EA[T FOOD.]

NOT TOO MUCH.

MAINLY WITH

PLANTS.

JEFF D LEACH

NEW ORLEANS 2008

Printed in the United State of America

For additional information, go to
www.paleobioticslab.com

Comments welcome:

e-mail jeff@paleobioticslab.com

CONTENTS

INTRODUCTION TO

EAT BUGS.
NOT TOO MUCH.
MAINLY WITH PLANTS.

This book is a personal selection from among articles, reflections and tirades that I have published – or in some cases not published – over the last 2 years. Though a lack of structure to the book will be obvious from the get go, my intention in compiling these "select" articles was to drive home some simple messages about the role of fiber in human health – a detailed synthesis on the science of fiber and human health *is not* the goal of this "little" book. As you bounce from chapter to chapter across the many themes I hope the redundancy of the message leaves a permanent stain on your future outlook on the important role of this carbohydrate – and the gut bug that rely on it – on the evolutionary success and future of our species. If not, at least the book has been printed on soft paper!

Jeff D Leach
New Orleans 2008

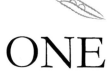

ONE

GUT CHECK[1]

The 2008 outbreak of Salmonella Saintpaul has drawn outcry from media, predictable knee-jerk proposals from lawmakers, and understandable fear and confusion among consumers. As with outbreaks in the past, the Food and Drug Administration (FDA), Centers for Disease Control and Prevention (CDC), and processing plants and farmers continue to take the blame for tainted food making us ill. But is our All-American sick gut deserving of some blame as well?

While our attention is focused on farm-to-table food safety and disease surveillance *once we have gotten sick*, the biological question of *why* we got sick is all but ignored.

---

[1] A version of this article appeared as an Op-ed piece in the July 28, 2008 issue of the *San Francisco Chronicle*.

Most experts working within what might be called the U.S. Food Safety System, that includes the efforts of some 15,000 people from 15 federal agencies, would readily acknowledge the complexity of detecting the admittedly small numbers of pathogenic bacteria and viruses in the 350 billion pounds of food in a farm-to-table chain that often spans multiple time zones and countries, as an insensitive prevention strategy at best.

Likewise, once an outbreak has been detected, sourcing the offending pathogen can prove difficult, as the ongoing Salmonella Saintpaul outbreak demonstrates even when a genetic match is made. While good farming practices, sampling and testing for detection, and the secondary prevention of tracking down the bad bug once an outbreak has been recognized are critical to a safe food supply, understanding why a person succumbs to what is often a very small number of initial organisms may be a relevant question and an additional strategy in reducing human suffering from foodborne pathogens.

By adding the *biological* question of why an individuals natural defenses failed to the *intellectual concepts* of testing, detection, and surveillance, we correctly insert personal responsibility into our national strategy and more importantly, draw attention to the much larger public health crisis, of which illness from foodborne pathogens is only a symptom: our sick, leaky guts.

The CDC warns "The elderly, infants, and those with impaired immune systems are more likely to have a severe illness" associated with tainted food (and water). By "impaired" the CDC is saying that within the complex network of specialized cells and organs that work together to defend against attacks from foreign invaders like Salmonella, something has gone wrong, increasing risk of getting sick – or worse.

A critical component to a properly functioning immune system is a healthy, and balanced population of bacteria. With names like bifidobacterium and lactobacillus, these and other natural inhabitants of the human gut make it their evolutionary job to fight invaders by competing for nutrients (which the invader needs to survive), compete for attachment sites on our intestinal walls (which the invader must do to cause harm), production of organic acids (that the invader does not like), and changing of pH of intestinal ecosystem (which the pathogen does not like either, but fast learning how to adapt). The things that are

This germ-on-germ warfare is literally fought daily in the American gut. When the good guys lose, we know this as diarrhea, fever, and abdominal cramps – or worse. We have all experienced or witnessed these lost battles at varying levels from being restricted to the house, visits to the emergency room, or in some extreme cases, the morgue. While this germ warfare has raged in the human gut as long as humans have been around, the rules of the battle are changing as humanity has started a large-scale experiment by shifting to a highly processed diet that has changed the nutrient supply that our friendly microbes evolved to depend upon.

The irony of the public running from vegetables and fruits that have been suspected in an outbreak, is that these foods contain essential nutrients (dietary fiber) that our gut bugs need to fight the good fight. Our change in diet, coupled with uncontrolled use of antibiotics, may be adversely altering our organic relationship with our most important weapon against foodborne pathogens.

The disruption and increased gut infections caused by pathogens is possibly having an irreversible impact on our entire gastrointestinal system. Like a siege of cannon fire on the walls of a fortress, the walls (barrier) begin to crumble (impaired) and become prone to invasion. Mounting evidence suggests acute and chronic infection by pathogens damage the delicate mucosa barrier that separates trillions of bacteria in our intestinal system from the sterile environment of our blood. As the steady flow of lost battles accumulate, the barrier and our immune system as whole become impaired, resulting in inflammation and movement of pathogens (and endotoxins) into our sterile blood. An impaired and leaky gut barrier plays an important role in a range of maladies such as irritable bowel disease, some cancers, sepsis, organ failure, heart disease and a cascade of other metabolic disorders.

By inserting personal responsibility and some basics of host-pathogen germ warfare into the multi stakeholder strategy for addressing foodborne threats, we may start to realize that we may not simply be experiencing a mathematical rise in foodborne illness as a result of sloppy farming and poor government oversight, but rather a tectonic like shift in our nutritional landscape that has opened the pathogens door just enough for us to glimpse the future of human suffering. Just the thought makes my gut ache.

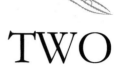

TWO

ARE GOVERNMENT RECOMMENDATIONS FOR DAILY FIBER INTAKE TOO LOW?[2]

Modern humans are the latest in a diverse line of species within the genus *Homo* that evolved on a nutritional landscape very different from the one we find ourselves on today. During the ~ 2.5 million years since the first member of our genus made an appearance in the fossil record, humans subsisted on an extraordinary diversity of wild plants and animals from a dynamic environment that

[2] An earlier version of this article appeared in May 2008 issue of *Network Health Dietitians Magazine* (UK).

literally changed at a glacial pace. It is only within the last 5,000 to 10,000 years that our food supply has begun to include domesticated plants and animals. For more than 99 % of human history, our genome and its nutritional and physiological parameters were selected during our non-domesticated foraging life-way conditioned, in no small way, by a diet that included large amounts of dietary fiber from a *significant diversity* of sources.

Even though this important reality underlies the basic evolutionary biological principles of modern human nutrient requirements, it is all but missing from policy and research discussions on recommended intake of dietary fibre throughout the world. Even more startling, much of our discussion on the health benefits of fibre, at least in the U.S. and U.K., often refer to the mechanical actions of fibre (stool bulking, for example) and nearly ignores the critical role of dietary fiber as a nutrient base of sorts for the trillions of microbes living throughout the human gut.

It's safe to say that our current chronic low-intake of dietary fibre in the western world (~12 to 15g/d) – coupled with our overuse of antibiotics and the increase in multiple antibiotic resistance in pathogens – has started a large-scale genetic "re-engineering" experiment on the slowly evolved and critical symbiotic relationship between humans and our little evolutionary hitchhiking friends, with limited discussion of its outcome on public health.

As you read this, there are millions of tiny microbes swimming around in the fluid surrounding your eyeballs. But you can't see them. There are millions more under your fingernails, on your hands, arms, legs and just about every imaginable section of your fleshy real estate. There are millions more lining your moist nasal passage, many more maneuvering about your liver, heart, lungs, pancreas and trillions more have been living throughout your continuous gastrointestinal tract – from mouth to anus – from the moment you enter this world. But this is good news.

The bad news is as we fill our shopping carts and pantries with the latest neatly boxed and wrapped goodies of industry, we continue down a path that began some ten thousand years ago with the emergence of agriculture – an event that eventually, along with steel roller mills in the 1880s, farm subsidies in the 1970s, and the divergent interests of food sellers and public health, may be leading us on a path to one of the greatest unintended consequences in human history by tinkering with the health of our intestinal microbes. Current dietary advice would be well served by an appreciation that the average human is a complex super-organism, rather than a single individual.

The archaeological and ethnographic record serves as an interesting reminder of the magnitude of the shift in the diversity and quantity of fibre in human diet.

Along the shores of the Sea of Galilee in modern-day Israel, a remarkably well-preserved collection of plant remains recovered from the 23,000-year-old archaeological site of Ohalo II provides an extraordinary window into a broad-spectrum diet that yielded a collection of >90,000 plant remains representing small grass seeds, cereals (emmer wheat, barley), acorns, almonds, raspberries, grapes, wild fig, pistachios, and various other fruits and berries. Owing to excellent preservation, a stunning 142 different species of plants was identified, revealing the rich diversity of fibre sources that was consumed by the site inhabitants.

In Australia, Aborigines are known to have eaten some 300 different species of fruit, 150 varieties of roots and tubers, and a dizzying number of nuts, seeds, and vegetables. Recent analysis of over 800 of these plant foods suggest the fibre intake was estimated between 80 to 130 g/d – possibly more – depending on the contribution of plants to daily energy needs. In semi-arid west Texas, a nearly continuous 10,000-year record of ancient foraging reveals a plant-based diet that conservatively provided between 100 to 250 g/d of dietary fibre. Analysis of hundreds of preserved human feces (coprolites) recovered throughout the 10,000-year archaeological sequence reveal a significant diversity of plants was consumed.

While the diversity and quantity of fibre varied spatially and temporally in the past, our ancestors clearly evolved on a diet that included daily intake of fibre from a huge diversity of sources that far exceed those recorded among populations in recent intervention and prospective studies concerned with the role of fibre in human health. These modern studies invariably group people with fibre intakes hovering around 20 g/d as the "high fibre" group, when in reality these high fibre or upper quintile groups are in fact low from an evolutionary perspective. Therefore, from an evolutionary perspective we should not be surprised when analytical hair splitting of these minute amounts of fibre does not yield the desired protective role one might suspect going into the study.

The potential protective role of dietary fibre among these modern studies may further be complicated by the lack of diversity as much as the quantity. According to data compiled by the Economic Research Service, United States Department of Agriculture in 2007, 57% of all vegetables consumed by Americans are limited to five sources (potatoes, tomatoes, leafy greens, lettuce, and onions). Unfortunately, the most consumed vegetable in America, the potato, is often in the form of oil-soaked french fries or potato chips. For fruit, five sources (apples, bananas, grapes, strawberries, and oranges) account for 71% of the total intake. From an evolutionary perspective, this minimal diversity, even when coupled with the handful of whole grains and beans/legumes consumed, translates into a striking shortfall in the physical and chemical diversity of fibre once consumed by humans and subsequently utilized by the hundreds of bacterial species that inhabit the human gut. We have changed the rules of the game between "us and them" in such a way as to possibly disrupt the organic harmony that evolved in this symbiotic relationship to a nutritional tipping point.

The emergence of prebiotics as a "super fiber" of sorts is just one example of the importance of diversity of fibre in the human diet. The steady clip of scientific papers demonstrating the health benefits of prebiotics is fascinating as we are literally peaking under the evolutionary curtain of our nutritional past. Unlike probiotics, which are live microbial organisms that are naturally present in the human body, prebiotics are literally food for probiotics. While many fibres claim to be prebiotics, true prebiotics selectively stimulate the growth of certain probiotics known to be beneficial to humans, such as bifidobacterium and lactobacillus, while not promoting the growth of less useful or even harmful strains, such as clostridium.

Even though prebiotic fibres are present in more than 30,000 edible plants throughout the world, American and European diets only include 1 to 3 g/d – sometimes a little more, sometimes a little less. When we look into the archaeological record, like the west Texas example discussed above, we see daily consumption (though variable seasonally) of 10, 15 and often more than 20 g/d from desert plants such as agave, prickly pear, sotol, wild onions and so forth. Dozens of peer-reviewed studies have shown that test subjects who consumed between 5 to 20 g/d of prebiotic fiber, mainly in the form of inulin and fructo-oligosaccharides derived from chicory roots, were able to stimulate the growth of "good" bacteria and increase calcium absorption, blunt hunger, relieve symptoms of irritable bowel syndrome, reduce biomarkers of some cancers, reduce inflammation through various mechanisms, improve immunity, and fortify our natural defenses against many food-borne pathogens. And the list goes on.

It would be a mistake to look at the science and health benefits emerging from clinical benefits of prebiotics as a *new discovery* of some magic bullet. More correctly we are simply witnessing a *rediscovery* of the importance of the diversity of fibre in human diet and, specifically, the role these particular fibres play in the health and well-being of gut bugs.

The exciting science behind prebiotics coupled with the underlying biological reality that humans are *still* designed to ferment a large and diverse quantity of fibre (~50 to 90 g/d, minimum), and that much of our health is tied to the maintenance of a healthy population of gut bacteria, should serve as a wake up call for new therapeutic approaches to health. We don't need yet another diet for us, but desperately need a diet for our entire "super-organism' – both us and them.

Even though humans evolved from nothing more than a run-of-the-mill large mammal on an open savannah of other large mammals, to something of a geological force in an evolutionary blink of an eye, we owe much of our current success as a species to these tiny microorganisms. They require little more than a safe place to live and a steady flow of the quantity and diversity of fibre that they and their microbial ancestors evolved on.

Continuing to ignore our shared nutritional past with our tiny friends and adhering to the very human-like notion that we are somehow separate from nature will only result in progression of many human diseases to levels that will require the medical community to seek new vernacular to describe the public health hardships that potentially lie ahead. Fibre anyone?

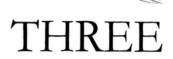

THREE

E. COLI AND THE FUTURE HEALTH OF AMERICA[3]

In 2006, Americans learned that a salad could be hazardous to your health. The media flurry and the elected official posturing that followed the September 14, 2006 outbreak of E. coli 0157:H7 associated with spinach, is still fresh on American minds and making daily headlines thanks in no small part to the brisk recalls associated with tainted beef throughout 2007.

So is our food supply less safe and are the growers, shippers, and various groups and agencies tasked with

---

[3] An earlier version of this article appeared as an op-ed in the SAN FRANCISCO CHRONICLE (January 22, 2007). A more recent version appeared as an op-ed in the agricultural newspaper THE PACKER, July 30, 2007.

oversight not doing all they can to protect the consumer from deadly microbes, as some believe? While the media and the public at-large lays blame at the doorstop of industry and government, might the brunt of this burden be misplaced? Simply, are we so involved in finger pointing, fences, and hairnets that we don't see the forest for the trees? An evolutionary perspective on the problem suggests, maybe.

Forgetting for a moment that the latest deadly microbe on the scene originates in cows,[4] one needs to come to grips with the fact that the microbes have us out numbered. When a handful of rich soil contains tens of millions of tiny microbes, and a single leaf of spinach may be covered in millions more, you start to get a feel for the germ warfare we are up against. Even worse, our so-called modern diet, which is dominated by highly processed grains and added sugars and fats, is putting us at a significant disadvantage in the battlefield that is us.

But evolution has equipped humans with an ingenious system for defending against this daily microbial onslaught, most of which are harmless. Our very own microbial foot soldiers, which set up shop in our guts the minute we enter this world. There are so many microbes in the human body that if you added up their total number of cells, they would out

---

[4] *Bovine Feces from Animals with Gastrointestinal Infections Are a Source of Serologically Diverse Atypical Enteropathogenic Escherichia coli and Shiga Toxin-Producing E. coli Strains That Commonly Possess Intimi.* APPL. ENVIR. MICROBIOL. 2005 71: 3405-3412.

number our human cells 9 to 1. In other words, we are more microbe than mammal.[5]

The vast majority of the trillions of bacteria that live in our gut, most of which can be found in our large bowel and represent hundreds of species, make it their evolutionary job to keep out the pathogens that seek to do us harm. In this complex bacterial ecosystem, potentially pathogenic bacteria (e.g., E. coli 0157:H7, Salmonella, Listeria) from the "outside" world are typically suppressed by a mechanism called colonization resistance. Since the human intestinal tract is a continuous system from mouth to anus, anything present within our gut is technically still outside our body. That said, a deadly strain of E. coli does very little harm as it travels through our gut, it's when it attempts to attach to the wall of our intestinal tract that problems occur.

In order for deadly pathogens to attach, they must compete for nutrients and colonization sites under a steady fire of microbial substances being hurled at them by our resident gut bugs. No doubt about it, this is germ warfare 101 and our gut bugs want to win. If our microbial foot soldiers are successful, then the pathogen cannot gain a foothold and consequently are swept from the system. If they are not suppressed, we quickly become aware of the lost battle from the all-too-familiar gut ache, cramping, and diarrhea, or even worse, death.

---

[5] *Evolution of Symbiotic Bacteria in the Distal Human Intestine.* PLoS BIOL. 2007 Jun 19;5(7)

This germ warfare has been raging in the human gut for as long as humans have been around. But recently, breath-taking changes in our diet have put us at a disadvantage. In order for our gut bugs to fight the good fight, they need nutrients and a critical component of that nutrient base is dietary fiber. By definition, dietary fiber is any part of a plant that cannot be digested and absorbed in the small intestine and ends up in the large bowel (colon). Once in the colon, dietary fiber is broken down and utilized by our good bugs for their own growth and turned into energy (calories) for us. This means, dietary fiber is not food for us but food for the trillions of bacteria that live in our colons. If you feed them, the bacteria will do their evolutionary job and make life a living hell for foreign pathogens.

Our modern genome and the symbiotic relationship we have developed with our gut bugs were selected on a nutritional landscape very different from the one we find ourselves on today. Our not-so-distant ancestors consumed between 50, 75 and often greater than 100 grams a day of dietary fiber per day.[6] The average American today consumes between 12 to 15 grams.[7] More importantly, our gut bugs

---

[6] *Evolutionary perspective on dietary intake of fibre and colorectal cancer.* EUR J CLIN NUTR. 2007 Jan;61(1):140-2

Institute of Medicine. Dietary Reference Intakes for Energy, Carbohydrate, Fiber, Fat, Fatty Acids, Cholesterol, Protein, and Amino Acids. 2002. Washington, D.C.: The National Academies Press.

[7] *Dietary fiber and the risk of colorectal cancer and adenoma in women.* N ENGL J MED 1999; 340:169-76.

evolved on a diet that included an extraordinary variety of fiber sources from hundreds of plants. Humans and our evolutionary hitchhikers went from a large quantity and diversity of fibers, to a small quantity and a limited diversity. We are literally starving our gut bugs to the point that we have opened the pathogen door just enough for E. coli 0157:H7 and its band of pathogenic brothers to compete successfully for nutrients and attachment sites. Not good.

The decrease in quantity and diversity of nutrient sources (dietary fiber) has created a nutritional tipping point in the germ warfare raging in the American gut. While increased oversight, inspections, sampling, and stepping up good agricultural practices are important; there are simply too many contamination variables from plough to plate. So rather than looking at the recent spike in outbreaks as a result of more pathogens in the food supply and sloppy farming, might the problem have more to do with our own dietary choices? That is, the breathtaking drop in the diversity and quantity of dietary fiber might be the real problem – or at least part of the problem. In other words, dare I say, there is some personal responsibility shouldered by the American public in this germ warfare.

When someone spends a lifetime smoking two packs a day, are they not aware that if they succumb to lung cancer, that it's, in effect, their own fault? So where is the personal responsibility in our national discussion on food-borne illness and the produce industry we seek to blame? Rather than running from spinach, let us run to it.

As the amount of dietary fiber in the American diet continues to decrease – probably even more so since last years' outbreaks – and our ignorance of the consumers' responsibility in this germ warfare continues, we may be seeing a perfect storm of our own creation – though unintended. The litigious atmosphere[8] surrounding this perfect storm has *already* created the potential for a public that sees diarrhea as a result of a nasty microbe as something akin to a winning lottery ticket. And the situation is likely to get worse.

However, the public's current mistrust of the produce industry may be an opportunity. Though tragic in its realization, the microscope the industry is currently under may provide a platform to explore some positive steps the industry might take in educating the public about how to increase their natural resistance to food-borne pathogens by returning the quantity and diversity of dietary fiber needed to support a healthy population of gut bugs. By consuming more vegetables and fruits, the American public may be able to add another weapon to our arsenal in our battle with food-borne pathogens and importantly, own some of the responsibility in this germ warfare. Currently, the consumer is totally unaware of the important role they play in keeping themselves and their family members healthy.

The produce industry does not need to wait until tomorrow to start this process, but start today. On September

---

[8] The Seattle-based law firm Marler Clark is emerging as the largest firm in the U.S. "dedicated to representing victims of food poisoning."

14, 2006 the produce industry stepped through a door and there is no going back. It's time to reposition produce in the American consciousness. The antioxidant and other micronutrient wagons the industry has hitched itself to in the past is tired, and the American public has been yawning at that message for years. The American public needs a reason to eat more produce, something new and fresh. Significant gains may be realized if produce is positioned more as fiber – that is, produce farmers are in fact fiber farmers. This "Fiber Defense Diet"[9] may in fact play a role in a much needed rallying call for produce in America and give consumers a very important reason to increase intake.

Some may suggest that the fiber defense argument for fighting food-borne pathogens is too simple, and therefore could not possibly make a difference. And they may be right. However, the human immune system and accompanying colonization resistance[10] mechanism that is facilitated by our own natural gut bugs makes all external attempts such as fences, increased inspections, and triple washing look like child's play. Our best defense has always been and will always be our natural resistance. Not nurturing our gut bugs with the

---

[9] See the Fiber Defense Challenge, www.fiberdefensechallenge.com

[10] *Dietary fructo-oligosaccharides and lactulose inhibit intestinal colonisation but stimulate translocation of salmonella in rats.* GUT, Nov 2003; 52: 1572 – 1578

Bifidobacterium strains from resident infant human gastrointestinal microflora exert antimicrobial activity. GUT, Nov 2000; 47: 646 - 652.

nutrients they need has consequences. Continuing to ignore this basic tenet of human biology will only result in an increasing number of our fellow citizens in the emergency room and decreased sales at the farm gate.

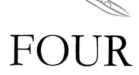

FOUR

C-SECTIONS, BREASTFEEDING, AND BUGS FOR YOUR BABY[11]

There I was, with a camera in one hand, wiping the tears from my eyes with the other. It was delivery day – I was going to be a dad. Like an eerie scene from a B-rated alien movie, out popped his little head from an amazingly small incision in my wife's lower abdomen. The

---

[11] A version of this paper appeared in MIDWIFERY TODAY MAGAZINE, Autumn 2006.

flash from my camera filled the room – this was the happiest day of my life.

Since that day over 13 years ago, my then-wife and I had another beautiful child, also through cesarean delivery. I had not given much thought to the fact that both my children entered this world through a small incision rather than the birth canal until recently, when the CDC's National Center for Health Statistics released its update on births in the US.[12]

Since my first child was born, the rate of c-section deliveries appears to have been rising at a steady clip, jumping over 40 percent since 1996. In 2004, 29.1 percent of all children born in the US were delivered through c-section – that's nearly 1.2 million incisions. The reasons for the increase are complicated, but have a lot to do with medical malpractice associated with vaginal deliveries, parental preference, health of the mother and, or the unborn child, and just plain old convenience.

In the days following the release of the CDC report, I scoured the media outlets that picked up the story to see if anyone mentioned an interesting and potentially alarming consequence of the rise of c-sections. I was looking for the mention of words human biology, bacteria, mammals, and the new nine-letter curse word of 2005 – *evolution*. Nary a mention from a single report – not one.

---

[12] http://www.cdc.gov/nchs/products/pubs/pubd/hestats/prelimbirths04/prelimbirths04health.htm

As a right of passage – a vaginal right of passage that is – the delivery of a fetus through the vaginal canal of the mother completes one of the most important cycles in the evolutionary history of humans. From an evolutionary point of view, our *sudden* adoption of c-sections as an increasingly preferred mode of child delivery may be tinkering with some very important processes that took millions of years to develop. Let me explain.

In what famed British 'Darwinist' Richard Dawkins calls an *evolutionary stable strategy*, humans have evolved a symbiotic relationship with a particular and complex set of bacteria in our gut. The 500 or so species of bacteria, whose numbers are measured in the trillions, occupy every inch of our gut – with most of them living in an ecological niche they literally carved for themselves in our colon. As the *evolutionary stable strategy* suggests, the presence of these few hundred species among all the tens of thousands of species of bacteria found in the air, water, and soil throughout the world that theoretically have access to our "open" intestinal ecosystem (think mouth to anus) is not random. This means our established intestinal ecosystem is composed of a set of bacteria that can live in nutritional and physiological harmony with us. Importantly, current members make it their evolutionarily determined job to keep out new members – i.e., pathogens that seek to do us harm.

The intestine of the unborn fetus in the mother's womb is sterile – devoid of any bacteria at all. However, during vaginal delivery the newborn comes in contact with bacteria-rich vaginal and fecal matter of the mother. These bacteria quickly invade and populate the newborn child. Saving of umbilical cords and the creepy ritual of eating the mother's placenta aside, this cycle links the co-evolution of intestinal "microflora" of the mother to the child, and may represent a more significant bond for those who understand it exists. This evolutionary bacterial right of passage has been and continues to be critical to the success of our species – and all mammals for that matter.

A child born through c-section essentially skips this critical evolutionary process. Though a c-section baby does receive bacteria from the mother, it's not the diverse and dense "base population" that it would have received from the vaginal fluids and fecal matter via a traditional birth.[13] In either birthing method, the baby is subjected to all the bacteria in the room – that even means the weird looking rubber-gloved fellow in the corner – who appears to be assisting the delivery staff in some way. But who can be sure?

Once this truly amazing and scary ritual of childbirth is completed, the newborn is typically cleaned, shown to the mother for short period, and then whisked off to some warm place to spend some quality time with other new members of our species. The mother usually settles in for some much needed rest and the new father anxiously paces the corridors mumbling to himself all of the things he is going to change or do better in his life. Seems some things are timeless.

---

[13] *Early supplementation of prebiotic oligosaccharides protects formula-fed infants against infections during the first 6 months of life.* J NUTR. 2007 Nov;137(11):2420-4.

But the next 24 to 48 hours pose another critical evolutionary step for mother and child – breast-feeding. Like all other mammals – and that includes our tree-swinging cousins – the secretion and release of fluid from breasts (mammae) is the sole nourishment or food for the newborn child. Yet, over 30 percent of new mothers do not breast feed in the hospital. It is often the case that some mothers never get their milk, others have problems getting the newborn to suckle, and others are just not interested.

At six months of age, the number of babies receiving breast milk drops to around 31 percent, and at 12 months it drops further to 17 percent. The number of babies receiving some level of breast milk at 24 months hardly makes a blip on the radar.

C-sections and short-term breast-feeding have no precedent in our evolutionary past. Before insurance companies and organized medicine, all children entered this world via the birth canal and participated in the time-honored cycle of transfer of bacteria from mother to child. Like our tree swinging cousins and a few of the modern forager groups that still follow traditional life ways today, breast feeding by the mother or other women in the group (wet nursing) continued for 24 to 36 months, sometimes longer.

Breast feeding newborns, like the evolutionary process of vaginal birth, is about bacteria. The breast milk of a human mother, like other mammalian mothers, is species-specific, having been adapted over eons to deliver *specific* and sufficient nutrition to guarantee proper growth, health, and immunity development. Researchers have long known that breast fed babies possess an intestinal flora that is measurably different than formula-fed infants. Of specific interest is a group of bacteria known as bifidobacterium. Some of you may immediately recognize the name, as they are often added to dairy-based foods such as yogurts – often advertised as "live cultures" on the packaging. These are probiotics.

Studies have shown that at one month of age, both breast-fed and formula-fed infants possess bifidobacterium but population densities in bottle-fed infants is one-tenth that of breast-fed infants.[14] The presence of a healthy and robust population of bifidobacterium throughout the first year or two of life contributes significantly to the child's resistance to infection and overall development of defense systems – not to mention the physical development of the intestinal system in general. Aside from the fact that substances secreted by these specific bacteria that are known inhibit the growth of pathogenic bacteria, they also work to make the intestinal environment of the infant more acidic, creating an additional barrier against invading pathogens. In short, breast-fed babies are sick less, are less fussy, have fewer and shorter duration of bouts of diarrhea, and have more frequent – and softer – bowel movements.

The dominance of health-giving bifidobacterium in breast-fed babies is due to the presence of special carbohydrates in

---

[14] *Dietary fibre and prebiotics in infant formulas.* PROCEEDINGS OF THE NUTRITION SOCIETY. Royal College of Physicians, Edinburgh, UK, 27-30 MAY 2002. 62(1):183-185, February 2003

mother's milk known as oligosacchrides. These special carbohydrates are virtually absent in cow's milk. From a physiological point, these special carbohydrates escape digestion and absorption in the small intestine of the infant, and thus reach the colon intact – where they serve as food for, among other bacteria, the all-important bifidobacterium. As the bacteria thrive on this "food" from mother's milk, they grow in number and absorb water, resulting in more regular and soft bowel movements. It's important to know that the bulk of infant feces are made up of live and kicking bacteria. Look next time if you don't believe me!

Baby formula manufacturers are catching on and creating products that contain these special carbohydrates – which are known as prebiotics (remember, prebiotics are food for bacteria and bacteria are called probiotics – see a few the next chapters in this volume). While it's virtually impossible to mimic the exact composition of mother's milk, it is possible to mimic some of the physiological effects – specifically targeting the growth of select bacteria through the delivery of oligosacchrides. One Belgium-based company (Orafti) in particular, has developed a natural variant of the mother's oligosacchrides from chicory roots (think chicory coffee). After years of careful study and peer review,[15] they are being added

---

[15] A nice overview of clinical research with prebiotics in infant formula: Boehm, G. and G. Moro, *Structural and Functional Aspects of Prebiotics Used in Infant Nutrition.* J. NUTR., 2008. **138**(9): p. 1818S-1828.

in greater and greater frequency to formula for infants. Any company that wants to stay in the lucrative baby formula business will need to adapt their products to include these ingredients, or else be left in the dust.[16]

In the dozens of doctor visits my wife and I made during pregnancy and through two births, never once did the doctor or any other person involved tell us what I just told you. In all of the "how to be a new parent" and "how to take care of your new baby" books we read, not one detailed reference to the critical passing of mother's microflora to the child via the birth canal or the importance of feeding bifidobacterium was ever provided.

In many cases, c-sections are absolutely necessary and should be performed. But a 40 percent increase in just the last ten years? This makes no sense. As a father of two, I am acutely aware of the physical and emotional toll that breast-feeding has on an active mother – the little creature literally sucks the life right out of you. Face it we live in a very different world than the one our not-so-distant ancestors occupied. Things are hard, but in different ways.

It's important that expecting parents understand some of the basic evolutionary processes of bringing a new member of

---

[16] For mothers who may not be able to breast-feed or must limit the time they do so, I strongly suggest you look into the exciting research on formulas that contain special prebiotic fibers (e.g., oligosacchrides). While its impossible to mimic mother's milk with formulas, some of the important physiological effects of fiber in mother's milk may be achieved with prebiotic fiber added to formula.

our species into the world. A few snips and stitches, followed by only a small number of sips, aren't going to cut it. The physical, nutritional, and metabolic features that make us uniquely human have been shaped by millions of years of evolution.

The debate in this country over evolution should not preclude health practitioners from understanding the *basics* of evolutionary biology. While we are culturally and socially modern, driving around in hybrid cars and arguing about stupid things, we are literally and biologically ancient hunter-gatherers. *Ignoring* our evolutionary past and its role in modern medicine and health, not just in birthing but also for ailments and diseases of modern civilization, is nothing short of medical malpractice.

Tinkering with or ignoring nature has consequences; it always does.

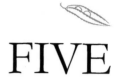

FIVE

PALEO LONGEVITY REDUX[17]

British nutrition researcher Geoffrey Cannon recently restated in the journal of PUBLIC HEALTH NUTRITION a widespread affirmation that "Paleolithic people usually did not survive into what we call later middle age." His underlying point, which is widely shared among researchers and the public at-large, is that our ancestors did not live long enough to develop cancer, heart disease and other chronic illnesses. All of which forms the basis for the

---

[17] A version of this paper was originally published as *Letter to the Editor* in the journal of PUBLIC HEALTH NUTRITION Volume 10, Issue 11, Nov 2007, pp 1336-1337

near universal belief that ancient hunter-gatherers (our ancestors) really were not healthier or fitter than us moderns, and therefore their ancient dietary practices have little relevance to modern health, well-being, and longevity.

On the initial point, Cannon is correct. The average life span of our ancestors was short, compared to that of modern humans in developed countries where one can expect to live into their 60s, 70s and possibly early 80s, on "average." Conversely, a Neanderthal living in ancient Europe was lucky to live past her teens, and if you lived to your mid-thirties you might have been considered old in Ancient Egypt. More recently, the average life expectancy in the United States in 1900 was 47.3 years. By 1935, that age had risen to 64 years and today that number hovers in the 70s for both women and men (though women can expect to live a few years longer, on average).

The first problem with this line of thinking is that the "average life span" math is misleading and tells us very little about the health and longevity of an individual, but rather gives us an average age of death for a given group or population. For example, a couple that lived to the ages of 76 and 71, but had one child that died at birth and another at age two ([76+ 71 + 0 + 2] / 4), would produce an average life span of 37.25. Using this methodology it is easy to see how one would come to the conclusion that this group was not very healthy.

However, the precept that diet played a significant role in the abbreviated average life span of our ancestors is simply not true. There are few among us that believe our so-called "westernized diet" of highly processed grains and added sugars and fats are an optimal diet for anyone – past or present. Our soaring rates of obesity and an ever-growing list of acute and chronic diseases – occurring in alarming frequency among younger sections of the population – speak to the discordance.

It is useful to point out that our species reached our current anatomical and physiological standing nearly 200,000 years ago.[18] That is, while components of what we discern as hallmarks of behaviorally modern human beings, such as language, art, trade networks, and advanced weapons, have only occurred within the last 50,000 years, the hardware has been in place for 150,000 years. While we may drive around in hybrid cars today, we do so in very ancient bodies and with a genome that was selected, for the most part, on a nutritional landscape very different than the one on which we find ourselves today.

Before the advent and widespread adoption of agriculture, which depending on where you lived occurred between 1,000 and 9,000 years ago, humans organized in highly mobile groups of dozens or a few hundred individuals. Archaeological data and analysis of burial populations[19] reveal that life was harsh and dominated by warfare, strife, destruction, human trophy taking, and the all-to-often practice of infanticide. All of these facts of ancient life, in conjunction with the lack of simple

---

[18] McDougall I., et al. *Stratigraphic Placement and Age of Modern Humans from Kibish, Ethopia.* NATURE 2005; **433**:733-736.

[19] Lawrence H. Keeley. *War Before Civilization.* OXFORD UNIVERSITY PRESS, 1996.

antibiotics and modern surgical practices, resulted in shorter average life spans than many of us enjoy today.

As agriculture took hold around the globe and groups settled down and built more permanent communities and ultimately socio-politically complex civilizations, the more homogenous and centralized food and water supply was easily contaminated by human waste. While war and even larger massacres continued throughout the agricultural revolution, tiny microbial killers took their share of victims, especially among the young and undernourished, further reducing the cyclical nature of the average life span. As European ships set sail just a few centuries ago, new ills and evils further reduced the average life span of populations they encountered – albeit punctuated.

As war, contaminated water, killer microbes, and illness pulsed through humanity over time, our basic underlying physiological and nutritional parameters have changed little in the last few hundred thousand years. Our modern genome is in fact an ancient one and natural and cultural selection has built it to last. Under optimal nutritional conditions, such as those our genome evolved on, us modern hunter-gatherers can live healthy and long lives. We need only look to the modern Hunza of northern Pakistan or the southernmost Japanese state of Okinawa to witness the longevity that our ancient genome is selected for. With the threat of war and violence greatly reduced, and upon a sound footing of a safe food supply, our ancient bodies can be healthy well beyond "our best-before date" Cannon writes about. Based on a low-calorie, high-fiber plant-based diet, a significant portion of the population enjoy healthy and active lives into their 80s, 90s, and often beyond 100.[20] Incredibly, the aged portions of these populations have lower rates of obesity, heart disease, diabetes, hypertension, high cholesterol, cancer, and other chronic diseases compared to western populations.

The modern world owes much to antibiotics and advanced surgical procedures of the last half-century, resulting in dramatic increases in average life span for much of the developed and developing world. Though horrific events in Darfur and other African regions remind us how significant gains in average life span can easily be erased. In Iraq, a male or female could expect to live to an average age of 66.5 in 1990, but today following years of foreign occupation and endless violence, life expectancy has dropped to a mere 59 for both sexes – and slightly younger for males.[21]

The self-confidence that comforts us today as we review the average life span of our ancestors is misguided and tenuous when viewed through the captivating haze of modern medicine that literally props most of us up into our golden years. I doubt our ancestors would call this living. While we may live longer than our ancestors, we are in fact dying slower. So rather than rest on our perceived cultural and medical success as it pertains to our longevity, we should challenge ourselves and our genomes to maximize our health for optimal longevity. For

---

[20] John Robbins. *"Healthy at 100"* RANDOM HOUSE, 2006.

[21] Population Reference Bureau. http://www.prb.org/Countries/Iraq.aspx. Accessed June 9, 2007.

those not trusting of the past and the nutritional landscape upon which we evolved, our genetic cousins, the Hunza and Okinawans, have shown us a way forward.

SIX

STRENGTHENING YOUR BONES

Osteoporosis. Just saying the word makes my bones ache. If you're a woman over the age of 50, you have about 40% chance of suffering from an osteoporotic fracture. That's higher than your risk of contracting breast and ovarian cancer. Even worse, 50% of the osteoporotic hip-fracture patients never fully regain independence and more than 20% will die within 6 months. Not good odds.

If you are someone who thinks osteoporosis is a "women's disease," think again. It affects 25% of men over the age of 50 and an alarming number of young people. If the current trends continue, the problem is expected to worsen by 60% in the next 20 years – regardless of gender.

Most folks are aware that osteoporosis is characterized by bone fragility and related to dietary intake of calcium, or the lack thereof. Simply put – calcium is used to build bones and to a lesser extent, teeth. From the time we are born until our mid twenties, our bones are continually growing and require calcium to do so. The goal during this critical growth period is to achieve peak bone mass. Thick, mineral dense bones.

Your peak bone mass – which again, you can only control until your mid twenties – will strongly influence your risk of osteoporosis later in life.

From our mid twenties to about age 50, the density of our bones is relatively stable. This means no matter how much calcium you consume, your bones are not going to get any denser. The goal now is to maintain the bone mass you developed in youth and minimize bone loss associated with aging. This is especially important for women, who must contend with a number of bone loss issues exaggerated during and after menopause – not to mention the demands of pregnancy and lactation on bone health.

While you are older and wiser, the efficiency at which your body absorbs calcium in later years, like some many things associated with aging, isn't what it used to be.

Despite the fact that we are confronted daily with the "eat more calcium" message for "healthy bones" on TV, in newspapers and magazines, on annoying billboards, and along the aisles of our favorite grocery store, nearly 70% of

Americans consume less than the daily recommended allowance of 1,000 mg of calcium a day – give or take.

Our daily intake may in fact be lower when you consider that, depending on our particular genetic makeup and the composition of a given meal, our bodies may only absorb 30-35% of the total calcium advertised for a given serving. Think about that little piece of critical information for a minute.

Calcium that is not absorbed is mostly excreted in our urine and feces, which brings up an important issue – and the point of why I am writing about osteoporosis – bioavailability.

The terms "bioavailability" and "absorption" are critical nutritional terms that are often used incorrectly. Absorption describes the process of transport of a mineral-like calcium from your intestine across the intestinal mucosa (the wall) into the circulatory system, so that it may be utilized or stored by the body. On the other hand, the bioavailability of a mineral like calcium means the "proportion" that is actually absorbed and thus utilized or stored.

The key here is solubility. A swallowed penny, for example, has zero bioavailability. It will simply enter one end and come out the other, intact. Whereas a glass of water is highly soluble and will be easily absorbed – nearly 100% bioavailability.

Even though you think you are getting 500 to 1,000 mg of calcium from a given food item, meal, or "supplement," you may not.

Given this piece of information, it's not only important that we increase our daily intake of calcium to recommended levels, we should also seek out means to increase the bioavailability of the calcium that we do consume so that it's not wasted, so to speak.

One way of doing this is to lower the pH of your gastrointestinal system by delivering food to the trillions of tiny bacteria that live in your colon (specifically lactic acid bacteria). And that means fiber.

Once in the colon, fiber is broken down by resident bacteria through hydrolysis and fermentation, which produces, among other things, short chain fatty acids and lactic acid. These acids then in turn make the colon more acidic, which increases the solubility of the calcium, making it more absorbable.[22] One of the short chain fatty acids produced (butyrate) has been shown to induce cell growth in the colon, which in turn increases the "absorptive surface" of the colon. This means more calcium is absorbed and less is excreted in feces.

Among the hundreds of species of bacteria living in your colon, you want to increase the number of the bifidobacteria and lactobacillus, specifically. These two particular groups are known to be especially useful in increasing the acidity of your colon – and they thrive well on special inulin and oligofructose-type fibers that occur naturally in onions, garlic, artichokes, asparagus, and in lesser amounts in wheat-based

---

[22] *Effect of prebiotic supplementation and calcium intake on body mass index.* J PEDIATR. 2007 Sep;151(3):293-8.

Diet, nutrition, and bone health. J NUTR. 2007 Nov;137(11 Suppl):2507S-2512S.

An inulin-type fructan enhances calcium absorption primarily via an effect on colonic absorption in humans. J NUTR. 2007 Oct;137(10):2208-12.

products. They are also commercially extracted from chicory roots (think chicory coffee) and added as a food ingredient in a growing number of foods. These special fibers are known as prebiotics.

By increasing the bioavailability of the calcium that we do consume through a more acidic colon, we can add an additional dietary measure to the preventive strategies for fighting this terrible disease.

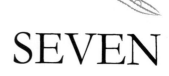

SEVEN

EAT BUGS. NOT TOO MUCH. MAINLY WITH PLANTS.

Why the FDA's plan to allow irradiation of lettuce and spinach 'may' cause more harm than good - but not for reasons you may think.

s of August 22, 2008, the Food and Drug and Administration (FDA) will allow food processors to irradiate iceberg lettuce and fresh spinach for the purpose of zapping E. coli and other pathogens. This ruling has been some time in the making and was recently fast-tracked due to the high profile spinach outbreak of 2006 and the pesky Salmonella Saintpaul outbreak of 2008. The FDA's

42-page ruling[23] predictably has consumer groups howling. Standard complaints and concerns run the gamut from "irradiation reduces the nutritional value of food, creates molecules unknown in nature, and changes the taste, color, and firmness of some veggies," to "irradiating veggies is just plain creepy."

The idea behind irradiation is simple: kill bugs. People in the produce industry call this a kill step. When you cook meat or boil veggies in your home you practice your own kill step, as microbes are pretty much terminated by temperatures above 140 degrees or so.

The Centers for Disease Control and Prevention (CDC) states that a little over 208,000 people a day suffer from some level of food poisoning resulting in diarrhea, cramping, and vomiting. Of these, roughly 5,000 die from complications associated with foodborne pathogens each and every year in the U.S. While many blame sloppy farming practices and poor government oversight for these numbers, our westernized diet of highly processed carbohydrates and low fiber intake may be more to blame.

In either case, consumers are losing confidence in the produce industry's ability to keep bad bugs out of fresh produce, and the industry views irradiation as the future of marketing 'bug-free' products to bolster consumer confidence. The consumer anxiety created by the high profile Salmonella

---

23 http://www.fda.gov/OHRMS/DOCKETS/98fr/FDA-1999-F-2405-nfr.pdf

Saintpaul outbreak of 2008, along with lobbyist-led efforts to change the law that requires food that has been irradiated to be labeled with the radura label[24] and carry the words "irradiated", replacing it with the much nicer sounding "cold pasteurized," is all but guaranteeing widespread adoption of irradiation – which will no doubt be promoted by government-backed consumer education programs in the years ahead with your tax dollars.

As fresh produce loses its innocence as it enters the irradiation era, nobody, including the FDA, USDA, or CDC, is asking what appears to be an obvious question: do we really want to kill 'all' the bugs on our produce? An eerily similar question was posed in 1945 by British bacteriologist Alexander Fleming, who discovered the antibiotic penicillin, when he warned in an interview with the New York Times that misuse of bug-killing penicillin could lead to mutant forms of resistant bacteria. Though nobody could argue antibiotics have not reduced human suffering since 1945, their overuse and misuse by the medical profession has created a terrifying list of antibiotic resistant bugs (think MRSA for example) that are killings tens of thousands every year in the U.S. alone and many predict will only get worse…much worse.

The lesson from Fleming and antibiotics – a 'kill step' that also has a friendly fire component (as antibiotics also wipe out all the friendly bacteria in your system) – is that panaceas for

---

[24] The Food & Water Watch website has a nice example of the radura label. Go to http://www.foodandwaterwatch.org/food/images/radura3.gif/view

public health may have unintended consequences. Deadly antibiotic-resistant bugs (though a predicted but unintended consequence) along with the friendly-fire wipe out of good bugs (though not predicted during Fleming's time but later realized and also unintended, which results in – believe it or not – overgrowth of unfriendly bacteria in the human gut following antibiotic treatment) may have a parallel in our national discussion to zap our fresh produce, which is loaded with millions, and often billions, of benign microorganisms. Their presence is a good thing.

To kill 'all' of the bugs on a leaf of spinach, as a casualty of friendly fire during the irradiation kill step aimed at the 'possible' contamination from an offending pathogen such as E coli 0157:h7, may have unintended consequences. Mounting research is revealing that humans are too clean and that this is in discordance with our 'dirty' past, which literally included being born in the dirt, living in the dirt, eating dirt at every meal, and so on. And we shared this dirty existence with trillions of microorganisms that lived in the same dirt and off the same foods we consumed – thus we consumed them. As a result, humans evolved a symbiotic and organic relationship with these ingested bugs to the point that our immune system has become dependent on them to operate properly.

Our national obsession with hygiene and removing dirt and the bugs from everyday life is giving rise to chronic inflammatory disorders such as allergic disorders (asthma, hay fever), some autoimmune diseases (e.g., type 1 diabetes and multiple sclerosis), and inflammatory bowel diseases (ulcerative colitis and Crohn's disease). It seems our immune system requires the presence of those dirt bugs to properly function. Without them, the system gets out of balance and overreacts to every little thing.

It was not that long ago that we ate fresh vegetables directly from the garden – minimally processed and no doubt covered in dirt and bugs. Those days are gone. A stroll through your local grocery store reveals neatly wrapped and packaged goodies from industry – all sterile and devoid of dirt and bugs, just what our 'modern' lifestyle ordered up. In the 1980s, the leafy green industry started triple washing produce – first a dip into some clean water, followed by a light chlorine bath, then another dip in fresh water. Got to remove those dirt and bugs! But microorganisms that make a living on the surfaces of our iceberg lettuce and spinach – newcomers to the irradiation club – don't give up their ground easy to a simple triple washing – hence the interest in zapping them (inside and out).

A child born in the U.S. today is likely to live in a sterile future. He has a fifty-fifty chance of being born via caesarean, skipping the trillions of vaginal flora of the birth canal – meaning he will spend the first few hours and days of his life without the benefit of his mothers protective bugs. This, coupled with the likelihood he will consume less breast milk than any previous generation in human history, means he will be endowed with an impaired immune system even before he takes his first step. He will spend his first few months and years of life not crawling around in the dirt and eating bugs as his ancestors did, but playing on indoor carpet and concrete playgrounds all under the watchful eye of parents who will quickly "wet wipe" away any signs of filth – catching the remainder in a nightly bath of suds containing antibiotic substances that will contribute to the antibiotic resistance of a growing menace. He will spend his days downing food-like substances boxed and packaged for maximum cleanliness. And when he moves from the nest and makes his own food choices throughout life, his cart will no doubt be filled with freshly irradiated produce – with no bugs – with a fresh-looking cold pasteurized label.

He will – quite literally – be the sickest generation of our species in human history, though you will not know it. Big Pharma will guarantee he makes it through the day.

Even though the relationship between removing dirt and bugs and the explosion in chronic inflammatory disorders, some autoimmune diseases, and inflammatory bowel diseases is the subject of countless peer-reviewed articles every year, nobody from the CDC, FDA, USDA and so forth has 'ever' come to the defense of the harmless bugs on the fresh produce we now seek to zap with irradiation.

Nobody doubts the good intentions of government scientists to improve the health of America, no more than we doubt the meddling of industry and lobbyists to influence those government agencies in directions that maximize influence and ultimately profits. This is how it all works, after all, through the system we support each election year. But lets not suffer from a failure of imagination. A little dirt and a few bugs might be just what the doctor ordered.

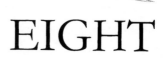

EIGHT

SO GO THE PIMAS, SO GO THE REST OF US

Anyone familiar with the American Southwest may have heard of the Pima Indians of south-central Arizona. The Pima are the modern descendents of the famous desert Hohokam who occupied vast swaths of south-central Arizona from roughly 200 BC to AD 1450. Famous among archaeologists for their massive and intricate canal systems built to deliver water to the arid and ecologically defiant agricultural fields of the parched Southwest, the Hohokam are a true success story of the ancient world.

While history paints the Hohokam as masters of their ancient environment, medical researchers fear our modern environmental landscape may be undermining their modern Pima Indian descendants.

In the 1960s epidemiologists started noting an alarming trend among the 11,000 or so Pima Indians living in the Gila River Indian Community just east of Phoenix, Arizona. For some unknown reason, a startling number of Pima were developing type 2 diabetes.

Diabetes affects tens of millions of Americans, resulting in the death of more than 300,000 people annually. It's also the leading cause of end stage kidney disease, adult blindness and amputation. The prevalence of diabetes among African Americans is nearly 70% higher than in Caucasians. Like obesity, diabetes dominates our national discussion on health care.

But for the Pima, however, type 2 diabetes and its complications are acutely devastating.[25] With the prevalence of diabetes estimated at 5.1% of the global population and 7.9% of the US population, the 38% recorded among the Pima of central Arizona gives them the distinction of being the most diabetes-prone group on the planet.

---

[25] *Genetic studies of the etiology of type 2 diabetes in Pima Indians: hunting for pieces to a complicated puzzle.* DIABETES. 2004 May;53(5):1181-6.

Once the trend started rearing its ugly head in the 1960s,[26] researchers saw not only a looming health crisis among the modern Pima, but also an opportunity to study the disease in a genetically 'pure' group, as many of the Pima married within their own community. Importantly, they had multiple generations within families in which to follow the development of the disease and the genetic predisposition. With millions in funding from the National Institutes of Health (NIH) and the blessing and cooperation of the Pima, the Phoenix Epidemiology and Clinical Branch of the NIH was established.

It is now several decades and 100 million dollars later, and researchers are still grappling with the Pima diabetes enigma.

So why are the Pima prone to diabetes? Diabetes research in general has determined that lifestyle (diet, smoking, physical activity, etc) and genetic factors clearly play a role. For example, there seems to be a significant correlation between ones weight and predisposition to developing diabetes and suffering from its complications. But among the Pima, given the genetic isolation of the group, it seems genes may play a major causal role in individual susceptibility. Or does it? A new study may shed some light.

If you happen to have been thumbing through a recent issue of the journal DIABETES CARE, you would have come

---

[26] *Preliminary report on the genetics of diabetes among the Pima Indians.* ADV METAB DISORD. 1970;1:Suppl 1:11-21.

across a fascinating study[27] by researchers who examined and compared adult Pima Indians of central Arizona with their genetic cousins, the Mexican Pima of northern Mexico. As mentioned above, the Pima of central Arizona are descended from the ancient Hohokam, who originally migrated to southern Arizona from what is today northern Mexico (several hundred kilometers to the south). Based on genetic, linguistic, and archaeological data, this migration is thought to have occurred a little over 2,000 yrs ago. Not all of the ancient population migrated and settled in southern Arizona, however. Some stayed behind to farm the highlands of Mexico. This situation has provided a unique opportunity for researchers studying diabetes and other diseases among the Pima of southern Arizona. On the one hand, you have Pima who have embraced the modern western civilization and its highly processed diet and lifestyle as it has swept over them, and on the other, you have genetically identical 'cousins' who essentially stayed on the farm.

The Mexican Pima live in remote areas of the Sierra Madre Mountains and enjoy few modern amenities. Many of these communities only recently became accessible by road. The Mexican Pima are primarily farmers and work manual labor jobs, such as those available in local sawmills. Almost every aspect of daily life includes physical activity.

---

[27] *Effects of Traditional and Western Environments on Prevalence of Type 2 Diabetes in Pima Indians in Mexico and the U.S.* DIABETES CARE 29:1866-1871, 2006

In contrast, the Pima of southern Arizona, who were traditionally farmers, "enjoy" a typical US lifestyle of computers and TVs, with low levels of occupational physical activity and lots of good ol' American fast and packaged foods. Those whose still farm have ready access to automobiles and mechanized farm equipment. Indeed, two very different worlds.

The researchers set out to test the following question by examining adults among the genetically similar but environmentally different sets of Pima: "Do type 2 diabetes and obesity have genetic and environmental determinants?" In other words, does environment (diet, obesity, physical activity, and other risk factors) play a role in the development of diabetes when the genetic pool is held relatively constant? If genetics played a major role in the southern Arizona Pima's astounding rate of type 2 diabetes, you would expect to see elevated levels in the Mexican Pima.

To add an additional variable to their study, the researchers also included Mexicans living in the same environment as the Mexican Pima in the Sierra Madre Mountains. The Mexicans (not of Pima heritage), are a mix of local Indians and Spanish. Like the Mexican Pima, the Mexicans live a rural and physically demanding life as farmers and ranchers.

Using Spanish-speaking interviewers and medical technicians, the data was collected. A brief medical history and physical activity questionnaire was completed on each participating individual, followed by measurements of blood pressure and a 75-g oral glucose tolerance test. The entire sequence was performed on 193 adult male and female non-

Pima Mexicans and 224 Mexican Pima near the town of Maycoba in the Sierra Madre Mountains of northern Mexico. In addition, obesity was assessed by BMI (weight in kg divided by the square of the height in meters), body fat was measured, and waist-to-hip ratio was determined. On top of all that, a 24-hour dietary recall was conducted to determine what everyone was eating.

Using the data collected from these two groups, researchers compared the obesity, diet and prevalence of diabetes to some 888 American Pima from southern Arizona. The prevalence of diabetes among the three groups is presented graphically on the facing page.

The prevalence of diabetes between the two genetically similar Pima groups is striking. Among the Mexican Pima men, 5.6% had diabetes, along with 8.5% of the women. Compare this to the Pima Indians of Arizona where 34.2% of the men have diabetes and 40.8% of the women. Among the non-Pima Mexicans (no shared heritage with the Pima), 5% of the women were diabetic and none of the men. That last part is worth repeating: *none of the non-Pima Mexican men had diabetes!*

In other words, age- and sex-adjusted prevalence of diabetes in U.S. Pima Indians was 5.5 times higher than their Mexican cousins and 16 times higher than the non-Pima Mexicans. The researchers also point out that the differences seen between the two Mexican groups was not significantly different (i.e., basically the same).

The differences between the prevalence of diabetes among the Pima Indians of Arizona versus the non-Pima Mexicans and Mexican Pima was also paralleled by differences in obesity, physical activity and diet.

BMI, percent body fat, waist and hip ratios were about the same among the two Mexican groups, but significantly different from the U.S. Pima Indians. The average non-Pima Mexican weighed in around 158 pounds (72 kg), with the average Mexican Pima at 145 pounds (66 kg). However, the average U.S Pima Indian male weighed 215 pounds (98 kg). While the women in all three groups weighed less, they followed much the same trend with U.S. Pima Indian females weighing, on average, about 200 pounds (91 kg).

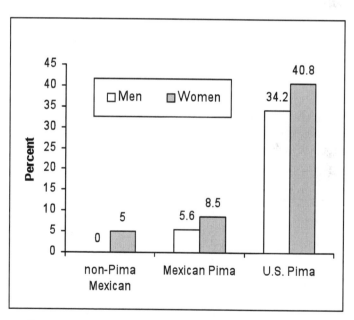

Rates of diabetes by gender across the various groups.

As you may have already sensed, the levels of moderate to heavy physical activity among the groups was higher for the non-Mexican Pima and the Mexican Pima compared to the U.S. Pima Indians. For example, the average U.S. Pima Indian women spent 3.1 hours a week on moderate to demanding physical activity compared to 22 hours per week recorded for her Mexican Pima cousin.

As for diet, nothing glaring jumps out between the non-Mexican Pima and Mexican Pima – other than a remarkably low percentage of calories derived from fat, ~25%. In the current study, the researchers did not collect dietary data on the U.S. Pima Indians. Previous studies, however, reveal that percentage of calories from fat for U.S. Pima Indians was much higher than the 25% recorded for the Mexicans groups.

The dietary fiber measured in the diet among the non-Pima Mexicans and the Mexican Pima's deserves some special mention. No matter if they were male or female, non-Pima Mexican or Mexican Pima; they consumed greater than 50 grams of dietary fiber a day. Compare this to the 12 to 15 grams a day the average U.S. Pima Indian, or the average American for that matter, are consuming.

Given the similar genetic background between the U.S. Pima Indians and the Mexican Pima, the nearly fivefold increase in diabetes among the U.S. Pima can only be attributed to differences in lifestyle and environments.

While researchers continue to look for genes that make someone of a distinct genetic group susceptible to diabetes and other diseases such as heart disease, the current study among the westernized and non-westernized Pima has taught us that obesity and physical activity have more to do with the likelihood that you will develop diabetes, regardless of your genetic makeup.

The take home message from the current study is profound: the genetic likelihood that you will develop type 2 diabetes is NOT inevitable and is CLEARLY preventable if you balance a reasonable amount of energy intake with energy expenditure and follow a diet low in westernized, highly processed foods.

However, the escalated levels of diabetes among the U.S. Pima and the increase of prevalence with age (for example, 77% of the U.S. Pima > than 55 years of age have diabetes) hint at some underlying genetic discordance with the modern food supply and environment. This is what keeps millions of tax dollars flowing into the genetic-arm of modern medical studies among the U.S. Pima Indians of southern Arizona.

I would add to the current study that the dramatic shift (drop) in dietary fiber in the U.S. Pima Indian diet from that of their Hohokam and earlier ancestors (who consistently consumed >100 grams of dietary fiber from a diverse variety of plants), has dramatically influenced the amount of insulin secreted throughout life, contributing to the metabolic condition of insulin resistance – a complication associated with type 2 diabetes. This metabolic condition, which I call *The Human Hybrid Theory* (see Chapter 10), potentially affects all modern humans who have shifted away from a diversity and quantity of dietary fiber that our ancestors once enjoyed and that our genome was selected upon.

It is worth noting that the non-Pima Mexican men, a group that recorded the highest consumption of fiber at 56 grams a day, not a single case of diabetes was noted. Not one.

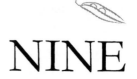

NINE

UNINTENDED CONSEQUENCES: WHAT HAPPENED TO THE HUMAN HYBRID?

A s you read this, there are millions of tiny microbes swimming around in the fluid surrounding your eyeballs. But you can't see them. There are millions more under your fingernails, on your hands, arms, legs and just about every imaginable section of your fleshy real estate. There are millions more lining your moist nasal passage, many more maneuvering about your liver, heart, lungs, and pancreas, and

trillions   more   living   throughout   your   continuous
gastrointestinal tract – from mouth to anus. And as you ponder
this unimaginable invasion of invisible aliens, there are millions
more setting up new beachheads on that all-important organ
between your ears every minute of every day from the moment
you enter this world. But that's the good news.

The bad news is we are literally starving, depressing and
killing off an alarming number of these little evolutionary
hitchhiking friends with our so-called modern, westernized
diet. Our modern food supply, with its 300,000 or so
processed products for sale in the U.S alone, is one stunning
example of the cultural, technological and political prowess of
a species gone wild. So freakish is our modern food supply, I
doubt our ancestors would recognize much of it as food at all.
Our internal 'friendly' bacteria are equally puzzled.

As we fill our shopping carts and pantries with the latest
neatly boxed and wrapped goodies of industry, we continue
down a path that began some ten thousand years ago with the
emergence of agriculture – an event that would eventually,
along with steel roller mills in the 1880s and farm subsidies in
the 1970s, lead to the greatest "unintended consequence" in
human history: The shift in how and where the human body
captures   much-needed   energy   (calories)   to   power   our
demanding bodies and lifestyle. Let me explain.

This admittedly dramatic pronouncement – "the greatest
unintended   consequence   in   human   history"   –   underlies
something I have come to call the Human Hybrid. The Human
Hybrid is an evolutionary-based way of thinking about
nutrition and the tragic epidemic of obesity and its growing list

of acute and chronic byproducts (disease). But nowhere is the Human Hybrid more potentially applicable than when trying to wrap your head around the metabolic syndrome of insulin-resistance (sometimes referred to as Syndrome X).[28] If you are overweight, diabetic, have hypertension, low HDL-cholesterol levels, high triglycerides, or have ever suffered a mild heart attack or stroke, then you probably have the insulin-resistance syndrome. More on this in a moment.

The easiest way to begin to explain the Human Hybrid is to think about hybrid cars – the latest must-have techno gadget for the socially and environmentally conscious among us. The concept behind hybrid cars is simple: a mixture of power technologies such as internal combustion engines and electric batteries (and in some cases electric motors) are applied to create a more efficient system. In other words, two power sources. On the front end you have a gas-powered engine that works to push the car forward part of the time, with the second power source (batteries) in the backend making up the difference a certain percentage of the time.

The clever engineers who devised the hybrid car designed it to run on both sources – not one or the other full-time. They share the work. Running the entire system on one or the other exclusively would result in the system malfunctioning and falling part. The two-energy system was designed to share in delivering the power needs. Like the hybrid car, humans have

---

[28] *Syndrome X*. CURR TREAT OPTIONS CARDIOVASC MED. 2001 Aug;3(4):323-332.

two major power sources – one in the front end (small intestine) and the other, quite literally, in the back end (the colon).

Our Human Hybrid is a hold over from our days of hanging out with other primates and enjoying those low-energy dense meals of roots, leaves, fruits, bark, seeds, insects, and flowers.[29] The good ol' days. Between 5 to 7 million years ago, the diet of our ancestors – who looked nothing like us at the time, and pretty much like our friends at the zoo – was dominated by lots and lots and lots of fiber. To extract enough calories from this bulky diet, our early tree swinging cousins relied on millions of years of co-evolution with an unlikely cast of microscopic hitchhikers and some ingenious arrangements.

As food passed through our early ancestors' stomach and small intestine, enzymes broke down the material allowing for fats, proteins, carbohydrates, minerals, vitamins and so on to be absorbed. Anything not broken down (fiber, and to a lesser extent resistant starch) was moved on. By definition, fiber is pretty much anything that escapes digestion and absorption in the small intestine and ends up in the colon – end of the line. Far from being wasted plant material at this last station in the gastrointestinal system, the trillions of bacteria that lived in our early ancestors colons went about the task of breaking down

---

[29] *Primate Diet and Biomass in Relation to Vegetation Composition and Fruiting Phenology in a Rain Forest in Gabon.* INTERNATIONAL JOURNAL OF PRIMATOLOGY, Volume 23, Number 5 / October, 2002.

Diet and Primate Evolution. SCIENTIFIC AMERICAN, 1993, 269:86-93

that fiber through a process called fermentation and turning it into energy. The bacteria relied on this "fiber" to live. In the process of fermentation, a byproduct known as short chain fatty acids, with names such as acetate, butyrate and propionate, were generated and then absorbed and used by cells and organs of the body as energy. *Voilà!* Energy (calories) from bark.

Rough estimates suggest that our early ancestors generated as much 25 to 35% of their energy needs by this hybrid energy technology. Primates living today still rely on the bacteria and the energy they generate to continue to make a living on the lush greens of the world's shrinking tropical forests.

As our earliest ancestors took those first tentative steps onto the open savannahs of Africa – and began their march to global mammalian dominance all those millions of years ago – they took with them this fully-developed hybrid energy technology and its bacterial power plant for the evolutionary ride. Today, this same cast of characters is still with us, known by names like bifidobacterium and lactobacillus (If you eat yogurt you will recognize these names as they are added today under the heading of probiotics).

But during that long march that ultimately ended in us, our diet improved as we explored new lands and developed technologies to extract more energy and nutrients from our environment. Over each new horizon, novel plants and animals presented themselves – and we ate them. We learned to fish, hunt, and to master fire – cooking food, making it more digestible and unlocking nutrients in quantities and diversities never before seen in primate-human history. And then within the last 10,000 years or so, pay dirt: agriculture, pottery, towns, cities, the wheelbarrow, Roman bathhouses! We never looked back.

As the quality and diversity of diet improved with every novel plant and animal we added to the menu, we digested and absorbed more and more energy and nutrients in our small intestine – the front power plant in our Human Hybrid. Through time, this resulted in an increase in the size of our small intestine to handle the windfall. Over the course of a few million years, our small intestine essentially doubled in volume – thus increasing the amount of energy absorbed in the front end. On the flipside, our colon (back end energy source), with its reduced role as a function of us eating less and less fibrous material, reduced in size by more than half.

Nevertheless, our modern colon still accounts for approximately 20% of the total volume of our omnivorous gastrointestinal system. Compared to the colon of meat-eating carnivores such as the wolf, it's downright huge.

The simple fact that the colon still represents a significant portion (by volume) of our modern gastrointestinal system speaks to its continued and important role in our Human Hybrid as an energy factory. If we did not need it to generate energy, evolution would reduce its size. Say, to that of a strict carnivore. Put another way: though our genome has evolved to less dependence on fibrous plant material through time, the fermentation factory – and its bacterial workers – is open for business today and will likely be so into the foreseeable future (a few hundred thousand years without a doubt).

So, 1,300 words or so later, you are probably wondering what this has to do with obesity and diabetes among the Pima Indians of Arizona or for modern humans in general. Quite a lot, actually.

Even though our modern colons still occupy an important place in our gastrointestinal system and our overall nutrition and the lights are on in the fermentation factory and trillions of bacteria (some 1,000 plus species) are standing at their stations waiting to do what they do best, our so-called modern and technically slick food supply and industrial and political landscape over which it flows have something else in mind – and fiber (food for bacteria and fuel for the backend power station of the Human Hybrid) isn't it.

By all estimates, modern humans should still be generating between 10 to 12% of our daily basal energy needs from the colon part of the Human Hybrid system through hydrolysis and fermentation of dietary fiber. For the average American or European who consumes a scant 12 to 15 grams of dietary fiber a day, the energy being provided by the backend is somewhere less than 1-3% - even less for some.[30] So how does this short fall translate into something tangible for or about modern human health? Quite simply, it means the front end component (small intestine) of the Human Hybrid is providing the majority of the energy demands and in the process, being

---

[30] Note this only considers the dietary fiber reaching the colon. Resistant starch, undigested proteins, fluffed cells and other substances flow nonstop into the distal bowel and may be fermented by the resident flora and converted to usable energy for the gut bugs and for the human host.

over worked – exactly what we do not want in a hybrid system of any kind.

The overworking of the front end is coming in the form of rapidly digested and absorbed foods that dominate our modern diet. This includes all those foods our ancestors would not recognize that are laced with added sugars, fats and highly processed nutrient- and fiber-poor grains (think sodas, ice cream, donuts, most breads, chips, *most* pizza and burgers, a lot of the dairy products, and so on). As we eat more and more of these front-end fuels, we are eating less of the backend fuel (fiber). The average American and European is getting nearly 60% to 70% of their total daily calorie needs from these front end fuels. This would be like pouring kool-aid in your gas tank and expecting everything to run the same as usual. Something has to give, and it is. Enter the hormone insulin and insulin-resistant syndrome – a root problem in a staggering number of modern ailments.

Since this important story needed to be told in such detail – hence it's length so far – I will restrict the remainder of the discussion to the development of diabetes and the role of the Human Hybrid (hang in there, almost done!).

The eating habits of our ancestors more or less adhered to the Human Hybrid diet that developed from the nutritional landscape on which our genome was selected. Our food supply consistently included up to and more than 100 grams of fiber a day – sometimes more, sometimes less. This meant our "minimally processed foods" contained copious amounts of slowly digested carbohydrates – an essential fuel for the red blood cells and brain, and the main source of energy for muscles under conditions of exercise (something that characterized everyday life for our ancestors).

For over 99% of human history (>2 million years), our ancestors main source of carbohydrates (primary energy source) were wild plants foraged from the ancient landscape. The sugars and starches (carbohydrates) in these plants were broken down by the enzymes in the mouth, stomach and small intestine (front end of the Human Hybrid) and absorbed into the blood stream along with other nutrients, and utilized by the cells as energy.

Plant parts that are, due to their either chemical or physical structure (fiber), not broken down in this front end of our Human Hybrid are moved along to the next energy station, the colon.

The most common and important of these energy sources is glucose – a building block of starch. Once glucose is absorbed into the blood stream, the pancreas jumps into action and excretes the hormone insulin that binds with the glucose and allows it to be utilized as energy. A cellular key of sorts. Without insulin, the glucose cannot be utilized. And this is where the problem begins.

Our ancestral diet was ideal because it provided slowly released energy in the form of slowly absorbed foods (today we know this as a low glycemic diet). This also helped to delay hunger pangs well after a meal and importantly, it was easy on the insulin-secreting cells of the pancreas and did not overwhelm the system with too much insulin or glucose. This system of gradual absorption of glucose and excretion of life-giving insulin was what our ancestors evolved on for millions of years and what our genome was selected upon. Like the very specific engineering of a hybrid car – which requires finely tuned inputs and interactions between components with everything operating just as engineered or else things don't function properly – our Human Hybrid was built in a similar Wikipedia-like way with slow and gradual shifts in diet over huge spans of time – evolutionary time.

Our recent adoption (mainly in the last 200 years, but more so in the last 30-35) and obsession with industry and government promoted "quick" energy in the form of easily digested and absorbed sugars and highly-processed grains, is throwing everything off.

When we start overwhelming the finely tuned Human Hybrid with too much glucose from highly processed foods, we are asking the pancreas to excrete more and more insulin at a faster rate. At the same time, we are also bombarding the cells in our muscles and organs with this never-ending flood of glucose and insulin at a rate and quantity never before seen in human history – something they were not engineered to handle. Asking the insulin-generating pancreas to put in overtime often (and usually does) results in it finally malfunctioning (lower insulin levels) or giving out entirely. Without insulin to bind with, the glucose stays in the bloodstream. We know this condition of too much blood glucose as hyperglycemia, or by its more common name, diabetes (type 1 diabetes, of course, is when the pancreas can no longer produce insulin).

Of specific interest to our Human Hybrid is insulin-resistance, which occurs when the normal amount of insulin secreted by the pancreas is not able to unlock the door to cells. To maintain normal blood glucose, the pancreas secretes additional insulin. In some cases, when the body cells "resist" or do not respond to even higher levels of insulin, glucose builds up in the blood resulting in the dreaded type 2 diabetes.

So why do the cells resist this much-needed energy? Like a sponge full of water, the cells are saying "enough!" – even when they are not full. Have they become exhausted from trying to keep up with all that insulin and glucose? The science says, maybe – most likely, yes. We know that our unfamiliar, rapidly absorbed diet is triggering some deeply buried genetic instruction to do so. In other words, the Human Hybrid is out of whack.

And for the Pima Indians of southern Arizona (Chapter 9), with the highest recorded rate of diabetes of any group on the planet, it seems to be "just a little" bigger problem. What in their evolutionary past – or more correctly, their nutritional past – predisposes them to this terrible disease over, say, a European? I think it might be in the "fine-tuning" or "final touches" on their Human Hybrid fuel system.

Up until about 10,000 years ago, all humans on earth were hunter-gatherers – making a living on wild plants and animals gathered about the landscape. No pottery, no agriculture, no animal husbandry. Pottery and agriculture first took hold in southeastern Asia, then the Mediterranean and then spread throughout what is today modern Europe. So over a period from 5,000 to 10,000 years ago just about everyone in Europe was making a living on a limited number of agriculture products and cooking pots (minus a few pockets here and there). For our Human Hybrid, this meant easier to digest grains – shifting from whole grains to minimally processed ones. And as the grains become smaller and smaller (think coarse flour) with each new grinding technology (mortar and pestle to hand stones to wheel stones and so on), the sugars and starches become more digestible and thus required "slightly" more insulin for these increasing levels of glucose in the bloodstream. So far so good, as the process was slow and gradual taking place over thousands of years.

But for the Pima of southern Arizona, dependence on finer and finer flours from cultivated grains occurred later – much later. Throughout much of the American Southwest people started dabbling with agriculture about 3,000 to 4,000 years ago – but it was not until about 1,250 years ago that it started to dominate the menu. This is thousands of years after it already took hold in the ancient European diet. And for the arid American Southwest, the recent agricultural grain diet was heavily subsidized by a broad spectrum menu that still included an extraordinary variety of wild plants – hundreds of species.

So while Europeans were starting to introduce more rapidly absorbed agricultural grains and seeking acceptance from the genome through making slight dietary adjustments (slow ones) to the Human Hybrid engineering (i.e., shifting more of the energy demands to front end – less fiber that is), our Pima friends were still clicking along on the same diet and Human Hybrid blueprint. They would not start to challenge their genome for thousands of more years.

On top of this, the Pima were latecomers to the pottery barn – only developing these handy cooking and storage vessels in any appreciable quantities about 1,800 years ago – thousands of years after their European counterparts. Pottery was a significant engineering change to the Human Hybrid as cooking heat and water make plant foods more digestible. During cooking, water and heat expand the starch granules, making them easier to digest and thus increasing rates of absorption, literally creating the world's first fast food.

So when you fast forward to today and level the playing field with our modern diet – everyone has equal access to the same technology and foods – the Pima may suffer just a little more because engineering changes to their Human Hybrid in the form of novel foods (agricultural grains) and technologies (cooking pots), genetic requests if you will, were introduced later in their evolutionary history. Thus, their genome has had less time to "try" (and I stress try) to adapt. On a metabolic level, this means when you a challenge a Pima Indian Human Hybrid system with more and more rapidly absorbed foods, their tissues exert a hyper reaction and become insulin-resistant just a tad quicker. This basic premise is similar to the issue of lactose intolerance – with some people who have been exposed to the lactose in the milk of domesticated animals for longer periods of time – suffering less from its effects.[31]

And one final note about the Pima Indians, their ancestors inhabited the arid lands of the American southwest for thousands of years, where the available edible biomass – both

---

[31] *Evolutionary genetics: genetics of lactase persistence--fresh lessons in the history of milk drinking.* EUR J HUM GENET. 2005 Mar;13(3):267-9

plants and animals – is dominated by fiber-rich plants such as the numerous desert succulents.

In other words, arid environments are dominated by plants and the plants are, as a function of their survival mechanisms in such settings, heavy on the fiber side of things – both soluble and insoluble fibers. In fact, when the ancestors of the Pima got around to growing corn, squash and beans on a large-scale about 1,250 years ago, they also planted fields and fields of the high-fiber desert succulent agave (agave is the same genus that is used today to make that delicious tequila!).

So if you squint just a little bit as you look back in time at the Pima ancestors, you see not the famous maize farmers of the American Southwest, but rather you see fiber farmers maintaining their Human Hybrid just as their ancestors had done before them and their descendants will need to do today if they want to break the cycle of disease and misery that a modern processed diet has brought to these people.

How's your Human Hybrid?

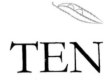

TEN

EVOLUTIONARY
PERSPECTIVE ON DIETARY
INTAKE OF FIBER AND
COLORECTAL CANCER[32]

F rom an evolutionary perspective, the ongoing
discussion of fiber's role in colorectal cancer is
possibly limited by the overall low intake of fiber
across study groups. Our ancestral diet consistently included a
diverse range of plants that regularly contributed >100 g/d of
dietary fiber. Importantly, this diversity assured that, due to a

---

[32] This paper originally appeared in the EUROPEAN JOURNAL OF CLINICAL
NUTRITION (2007) **61,** 140–142. Though more technical than the other
chapters in this book, it was written for a "general" science crowd.

range of physical and chemical structures, a steady flow of fermentable substrates promoted metabolic activity into the distal regions of the colon.

Modern humans are the latest in a diverse line of species within the genus *Homo* that evolved on a nutritional landscape very different from the one in which we find ourselves today. During the two million years since the first member of our genus made an appearance in the fossil record, humans subsisted on foraged wild plants and animals from a dynamic environment that literally changed at a glacial pace. Only within the last 5,000 to 10,000 years did that food supply include agricultural crops, domesticated animals, and their byproducts. Therefore, the modern human genome and its nutritional and physiological parameters were selected during our non-domesticated foraging life conditioned, in no small way, by a diet of *diverse* fibre- and nutrient-rich plants and lean meats.

Even though this important reality underlies the basic evolutionary biological principles of modern human nutrient requirements, it is all but missing from current discussions of dietary fibre intake and our attempts to understand its role in the etiology of colorectal cancer. As the steady stream of European and US-based studies demonstrate,[33] the protective

---

[33] *Dietary Fiber and the Risk of Colorectal Cancer and Adenoma in Women.* NEW ENGLAND JOURNAL OF MEDICINE, 1999, 340, 169-176.
Dietary fibre in food and protection against colorectal cancer in the European Prospective Investigation into Cancer and Nutrition (EPIC): an observational study. LANCET 2003, 361, 1496-1501.
Dietary fiber intake and risk of colorectal cancer: a pooled analysis of prospective cohort

role of dietary fibre is inconsistent, often frustrating, and made more elusive with a growing list of confounding risk factors (e.g., smoking, alcohol, red meat). This is further complicated when well-known fibre sources, such as resistant starch and inulin-type fructans, are not consistently considered when calculating total fibre intake amongst many studies.

Part of the dilemma in our ability to derive clear answers to the possible role of dietary fibre in colorectal cancer may be, from an evolutionary perspective, the remarkably low intake of fibre among various populations and study groups – even for those that fall within the upper quintiles. It is well known that dietary habits among westernized societies are characterized by increasing caloric intake from added sugars, fats, and highly processed nutrient- and fibre-poor grains. This caloric shift is in discordance with our evolutionary past[34] and continues to be at the expense of dietary diversity and consumption of fibre- and nutrient-rich plants. A few examples from the archaeological and ethnographic record demonstrate the magnitude of this shift as it pertains to the diversity and quantity of fibre in the human diet.

Located along the shores of the Sea of Galilee in modern-day Israel, a remarkably well-preserved collection of plant remains were recovered from the 23,000-year-old

studies. JOURNAL OF AMERICAN MEDICAL ASSOCIATION, 2005, 14, 2849-57.

[34] *Evolutionary Health Promotion.* PREVENTIVE MEDICINE, 2002, **34**, 109-118.

archaeological site of Ohalo II.[35] Ohalo II has provided an extraordinary window into a broad spectrum diet that yielded a collection of >90,000 plant remains representing small grass seeds, cereals (emmer wheat, barley), acorns, almonds, raspberries, grapes, wild fig, pistachios, and various other fruits and berries. Owing to excellent preservation, a stunning 142 different species of plants were identified, revealing that the site inhabitants consumed a rich diversity of fibre sources.

In Australia, Aborigines are known to have eaten some 300 different species of fruit, 150 varieties of roots and tubers, and a dizzying number of nuts, seeds, and vegetables.[36] Based on the analysis of over 800 of these plant foods, the fibre intake was estimated between 80 to 130 g/d, depending on the contribution of plants to daily energy needs. This daily intake is most likely higher when you consider that fibre in the form of resistant starch and oligosaccharides were not measured by the researchers among the economically important roots and tubers.

In the semi-arid Trans-Pecos region of west Texas, a nearly continuous 10,000-year record of a foraging lifestyle has been documented in dry cave deposits. Considered one of the most complete records of foraging lifestyle in North America, nearly three decades of excavation and extensive analysis of well-preserved macro botanical remains and human coprolites

---

[35] *The broad spectrum revisited: evidence from the plant remains.* PROCEEDINGS OF THE NATIONAL ACADEMY OF SCIENCES, 2004, **101**, 9551-9555.
[36] *Australian Aboriginal plant foods: a consideration of their nutritional compositional and health implications.* NUTRITION RESEARCH REVIEWS, 1998, **11**, 5–23.

(feces) from a number of cave sites[37] reveal a plant-based diet that conservatively provided between 150 to 250 g/d of dietary fibre from dozens of plant species. The fiber-rich diet is well illustrated by the visual presence of undigested fiber (cellulose) in nearly 100% of the human coprolites studied throughout the entire 10,000-year sequence.

While the diversity and quantity of fibre varied spatially and temporally in the past, our ancestors clearly evolved on a diet that included daily intake of fibre from a diversity of sources that far exceed those recorded among populations in recent intervention and prospective studies concerned with the protective role of fibre against colorectal cancer. While stool bulking, dilution of colonic contents, and reduced transit time are clearly positive mechanisms of this ancestral intake of fibre, of particular interest may be the increased opportunities for consumption of long chain molecules (e.g., inulin), in combination with insoluble fibres (e.g., cellulose, hemicellulose), that are known to slowly and selectively stimulate anaerobic bacterial fermentation into more distal areas of the colon. The slow, sustained effect of metabolic activity and production of SCFA (specifically butyrate), and corresponding reduction in pH and conversion of bile acids

---

[37] *Paleonutrition of the Lower Pecos region of the Chihuahuan Desert.* In PALEONUTRITION: THE DIET AND HEALTH OF PREHISTORIC AMERICANS, ed. KD Sobolik, pp 247 – 264. Center for Archaeological Investigations: Occasional Paper No. 22.

into more distal regions has been shown to have a strong physiological impact in biomarkers.[38]

With modern palates that trend towards less lignified portions of plants, in combination with a food industry that is likely to select added fibres more for their technical or economical characteristics than physiological ones,[39] modern populations 'most likely' consume more rapidly fermented fibres over more slowly fermented ones than at any point in our evolutionary past. Said differently, rapid technological advances within food industry and a decreasing variety and quantity of fibre sources throughout much of western civilization, has resulted in decreased metabolic and physiological activity in the distal colon, thus opening the pathogenic door to cancer in this region.

Future studies on the protective role of dietary fibre against colorectal cancer may benefit from a research agenda that includes an overarching understanding of the evolutionary landscape in which our current nutrient requirements were selected. In the case of even the best-designed intervention or prospective study, clear and optimal results may never be achieved as the diet and lifestyle of participants may differ significantly from their evolution-based and thus genetically determined optimal intake of fibre and other nutrients.

---

[38] *The specificity of the interaction with intestinal bacterial fermentation by prebiotics determines their physiological efficacy.* NUTRITION RESEARCH REVIEWS, 2004, **17**, 89-98.
[39] *Dietary fiber as a versatile food component: an industrial perspective.* MOLECULAR NUTRITION FOOD RESEARCH, 2005, **49**, 421-535.

Until we have better understanding of the diversity and quantity of fermentable substrates that entered our ancestral bowels and thus conditioned our current nutritional parameters and physiological responses, accompanied with modern analytical tools and techniques that allow us to compare the range of chemical and physical fibres present in the modern food supply, the possibly important protective role of fibre in etiology of colorectal cancer may not be forthcoming.

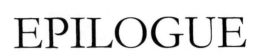

EPILOGUE

DO WE HAVE A FIBER CRISIS IN AMERICA?

After reading through the various chapters in this "little" book it should be clear that fiber is, well, uh…important. But it is important for reasons that maybe you were unaware of until now: fiber is food for bacteria, and these bacteria play an important role in our health and well-being. For those of us seeking better health and reduced risk of acute and chronic ailments, moving beyond the oft-cited decrees like "fiber is *Natures Broom*" will be required. This bizarre notion that fiber somehow sweeps the gut of all that is bad and toxic dominates much of our national discussion on fiber and highlights how little we all know about fiber and our health – much less the health of our gut bugs. Though there is an inkling of mechanical truth in that understanding of fiber, it misses the evolutionary, biological, and scientific importance of this carbohydrate.

It's safe to say that our current low intake of dietary fiber in America (~12 to 15 grams a day), coupled with our overuse of antibiotics and subsequent increase in multiple antibiotic resistance in pathogens, has started a large-scale genetic "re-engineering" experiment on the slowly evolved and critical symbiotic relationship between humans and our evolutionary hitchhiking friends, with limited understanding and discussion of its outcome on human health.

So where do our current recommendations on the amount of fiber we should eat come from anyway? Who determined this 25 to 38 grams a day range and why? Why isn't it less...or more?

As discussed in various chapters in this book, our current intake and the current recommendations of 25 to 28 grams a day are low from an evolutionary perspective and clearly low from the point of view of our gut bugs, who depend on this nutrient base. If Americans currently consume half of what the government recommends today, what if the government doubled those recommendations? Would we eat more and possibly get a little closer to the levels we need to achieve optimal health of our gut bugs and us – as well – in the process?

If people actually knew what fiber was and that it played a critical role in the health of our gut bugs (whom, if well-fed, play an often important role in the etiology of many diseases such as heart disease, many bowel cancers, inflammatory bowel disease and an equally important role in mineral absorption, resistance against food-borne pathogens and obesity…and the list goes on) might we eat just a few more servings?

Consumers are getting the message – albeit slowly – about the health benefits of gut bugs through the marketing efforts of yogurt products such as Dannon Activia® that contain probiotics. These products have done wonders for consumer awareness that "not all bugs are bad" and some are, indeed, good for you. They promise to deliver billions of live cultures (probiotics) with each sugar-laden cup of goodness. However, not all probiotic products are as effective as they would have you believe.[40] More importantly, why in the hell are we attempting to "replenish" or "fortify" our gut bugs in the first place? Many probiotic yogurt products contain one billion or more organisms. At first glance that seems like an astounding number of gut bugs – so the product must be good! Not so impressive when you consider that a billion probiotic organisms would barely cover an area the size of the "period" at the end of this sentence or that just one gram of your last stool sample contained possibly trillions of organisms. Rather than try to fortify or replenish, simply feed the ones that are already in your system the nutrients (fiber) they need. In the long run, you will not only feel better and be healthier, but you will save a ton of money on quick- fix probiotic yogurts.

The current message to consume more fiber is simply not working. As a recent survey has shown, it's not due to the lack of awareness of the importance of eating 5 or more servings a day of fruit and vegetables and getting a few more servings of

---

[40] http://www.guardian.co.uk/food/Story/0,,1839269,00.html

whole grains.[41] People hear the message – they get it – they just don't act on the message in a consistent manner.

Despite years of efforts by government, commercial interests, and non-profits to get Americans to consume more fruits and vegetables, only one in five Americans consumes the minimum of the 5 to 13 servings now recommended. Though adults are eating few fruits and vegetables, the trend is more troubling among kids. French fries were the most commonly consumed vegetable for children ages 12 to 24 months and "fried potatoes" (which includes french fries) make up 46% of the vegetables consumed by kids 2 to 19 years old.[42] On any given day, 45% of children eat no fruit, and 20% eat less than one serving of vegetables. Why do we continue to yawn at the health message to consume more fiber? If we shifted the message to focus on fiber as a diet for our gut bugs rather than a macronutrient for us, might folks eat more?[43]

Ask any one of the 67,000 plus Registered Dietitians in this country how much fiber you should be eating every day, and you will likely get the stock answer of 25 to 38 grams. Their

---

[41] State of the Plate: Study on America's Consumption of Fruits and Vegetables, Produce for Better Health Foundation, 2003.

[42] *FITS: Feeding infants and toddlers study: what foods are infants and toddlers eating?* J AM DIET ASSOC 2004; 104:S22-S30.

NCHS 2000. National Center for Health Statistics, U.S. Department of Health and Human Services. National Health and Nutrition Examination survey III. Washington, D.C.

[43] See the Fiber Defense Challenge www.fiberdefensechallenge.com

rapidly delivered answer will be based on a "position paper"[44] developed by the American Dietetic Association (ADA)[45] – circulated via the ADA's in-house journal and newsletters to its nation-wide membership of RD's. This massive army of nutritional foot soldiers marches under the following banner:

> "The American Dietetic Association is the nation's largest organization of food and nutrition professionals. ADA serves the public by promoting optimal nutrition, health, and well-being. *ADA members are the nation's food and nutrition experts*, translating the science of nutrition into practical solutions for healthy living." [Emphasis mine]

The ADA's position on daily intake of fiber mirrors the current *Dietary Guidelines for Americans,* which form the basis of the USDA's new snazzy Food Pyramid.[46] The ADA's current position on recommended daily intake of fiber was adopted in 2002 but expired December 31, 2007.[47] The *Dietary Guidelines for Americans* and accompanying Food Pyramid are due for revision on or about 2010.

---

[44] *Health Implications of Dietary Fiber.* JOURNAL OF THE AMERICAN DIETETIC Association 2002; 102:993-1000.

[45] The ADA's official website is www.eatright.org

[46] http://www.mypyramid.gov/

[47] According to the ADA, a new "white paper" on dietary fiber intake will be published sometime in 2008.

Ask this same question – "how much fiber should I be consuming on a daily basis?" – of a research-oriented gut microbiologist from any one of the leading research labs scattered throughout the world, who specializes in the physiological role of dietary fiber in the human gastrointestinal system and its role in the health of our microflora, and you will first receive the qualifier that fiber really means fermentable substrates and then you will be given an answer that hovers around 100 to 150 grams a day – possibly more, depending not so much on your chromosomes, age, and whether you take the stairs everyday, but on what kind of fiber you are talking about.[48]

The microbiologists' answer will also be rapidly delivered and based on a well-informed understanding of what fiber is: an important nutrient (carbon source) for bacteria that live in your gut (mostly your colon), and thousands of peer-reviewed articles, books, and massive ongoing research projects underway throughout the world. You will not hear much talk about *Natures Broom*.

Ask this same question yet again, but of an anthropologist who studies ancient dietary patterns of our not-so-distant ancestors, and you will likely get an answer of 50, 75, and up to 150 grams a day – possible more – depending on season, geographical location, technology available, and chronological period. This answer, which will not be rapidly delivered but

---

[48] Even though there are thousands upon thousands of variations of fiber, the top fibers used by the food industry in America are known by names like carragenan, xanthan, and guar gum – never mind if you don't know what these are, nobody else does either.

will be soaked in some history lesson that will drag on forever, will be based on evidence from analysis of plants remains from ideal contexts, such as dry caves, ethnographic accounts, the analysis of fossilized human feces, and from carbon and stable isotope analysis of skeletal bones from these same ancestors (cross-referenced with a dizzying array of other analysis from study sites all over the world). Man the hunter is more correctly man the gatherer. *Veggies, It's What's for Dinner.*

So how and why does each of these groups arrive at such different recommendations? More interestingly, why do the recommendations of the 67,000 dietitians informed by the US Dietary Guidelines and Food Pyramid differ so much from that of the microbiologist and anthropologist, which essentially overlap?

Based on our current intake of fiber, if you are following the recommendation of RD's and the US Food Pyramid, you are getting less than half to one third of the amount of fiber you should be consuming. From a microbiological and anthropological point of view, you are possibly eating less than 5 to 10% of the fiber that you physiologically require and that our ancestors regularly consumed (what our gut bugs need).

The RD's and the US Food Pyramid goals are an outgrowth of opinion by a panel of experts (congress and the USDA employees) informed by a report issued by THE FOOD AND NUTRITION BOARD, as part of the INSTITUTE OF MEDICINE OF THE NATIONAL ACADEMY OF SCIENCES. In this massive report[49] in 2002 to Congress and the USDA, these experts culled the scientific literature to come up with the

---

[49] http://www.iom.edu/CMS/3708.aspx

"very best" recommendations they could for nutritional parameters for Americans – based solely on the "best science available."

In other words, the U.S. Food Pyramid relies on this report for its design and overall justification (or lack thereof) for recommended daily intakes of the various macro- and micronutrients that our current food chain has been unfortunately broken down into.

In this massive report, located in the chapter titled *Dietary, Functional, and Total Fiber* – the chapter used to "set" how much fiber we should be eating – the authors state "An Adequate Intake (AI) for *Total Fiber* in foods is set at 38 and 25 g/d for young men and women, respectively, based on intake level observed to protect against coronary heart disease." This means, based on a handful of studies the report cite on heart disease and fiber, current recommended intakes are based on how fiber relates to *this particular* malady; gut bugs are not mentioned. The authors go on to say – interestingly – "There was insufficient evidence to set a Tolerable Upper Intake Level (UL) for *Dietary Fiber* or *Functional Fiber*. Again, translation: Even though the expert panel recommends that 25 to 38 grams a day should cover it, there is no data that says you should not consume more.

However, the expert panel seems to lean on a simple misunderstanding to limit the intake of fiber to 25 to 28 grams a day. You will often hear health professionals parroting this concern as well: that eating too much fiber *might* reduce the bioavailability of some minerals such as iron, calcium, and zinc.[50] What they are getting at are a limited number of studies

---

[50] *Fiber, phytates, and mineral nutrition.* NUTR REV 1992. 50:30-31

that have shown that when fibers that include phytate are present, malabsorption of some minerals has been shown. This is true. However, phytic acid is only present in appreciable quantities in the outer coating (bran, the fibrous outer coating of the grain) of some commonly eaten cereal grains but rarely or minimally present in most vegetables and fruits. The report fails to mention this critical little point. It seems strangely odd that an effect caused by consuming some grains and not veggies *per se* should be used to limit our intake of fiber.

Consequently, a diet high in fiber based on vegetables and fruits (and legumes) would have little or no effect on mineral absorption. And, as pointed out in Chapter 6, increased consumption of some dietary fiber *will actually increase* mineral absorption!

The story of fiber in human diet and health is a long one. We would all do well to ask more questions as individuals about this critical carbohydrate. The current message of fiber in our diet is honestly out-dated. The exciting science behind fiber and its role in the health and well being of our gut bugs is opening a new chapter in nutritional sciences and medicine. So pay a little more attention to the health of your tinny little friends within, and feed them. And the best way to do that is articulated nicely by author Michael Pollan: *Eat food. Not too much. Mostly plants.*

A FEW HIGH
FIBER RECIPES

In no particular order

TUSCAN TUNA SALAD
Prep: 20 min.

1/2 head Romaine lettuce
13 ounces marinated artichoke hearts, cut in half, marinade reserved
3 Tbs. balsamic vinegar
2 tsp. packaged pesto sauce
2 lbs. canned Great Northern beans, drained and rinsed
1/4 lb. sun-dried tomatoes, prepared according to package directions
1/3 cup black olives
13 ounces canned water-packed albacore tuna, flaked

Line a platter with lettuce leaves. Combine reserved artichoke marinade, vinegar and pesto in a bowl. Add artichokes, beans, tomatoes and olives. Toss gently and spoon over lettuce. Top with tuna and drizzle with any remaining dressing from bowl. Serve at room temperature.

PER SERVING: calories 574, fat 12.4g, 18% calories from fat, cholesterol 28mg, protein 49.6g, carbohydrates 73.7g, **fiber 24.7g**, sugar 16.7g, sodium 1519mg

ITALIAN BEAN AND TUNA SALAD
Prep: 15 min, plus refrigeration time

11 ounces canned baby lima beans, rinsed, drained
11 ounces canned dark red kidney beans, rinsed, drained

10 ounces canned Great Northern beans, rinsed, drained
5-1/4 cherry tomatoes cut into fourths
1/4 small cucumber, cut lengthwise into halves, seeded, sliced
3-1/2 Tbs. green or red bell pepper, chopped
1/4 red onion, thinly sliced
2 Tbs. olive oil
1/3 cup tarragon white wine vinegar
1 tsp. dried basil leaves
2 Tbs. nonfat plain yogurt
1 Tbs. lemon juice
1/2 tsp. sugar
1 Tbs. water
2 cloves garlic
11 ounces tuna steak, broiled or grilled, or canned white tuna
in water, drained, flaked into small pieces
5-1/4 large lettuce leaves
2-3/4 basil or parsley sprigs

Combine beans, tomatoes, cucumber, pepper, and onion in
large bowl. Add the next 8 ingredients (basil vinaigrette) and
toss. **Refrigerate** mixture at least 4 hours for flavors to blend,
stirring mixture occasionally. Add tuna to mixture 1 to 2 hours
before serving. Spoon salad onto lettuce-lined plate; garnish
with basil.

You can make the bean salad one day in advance and
refrigerate, adding tuna 1 to 2 hours before serving.

PER SERVING: calories 454, fat 9.1g, 18% calories from fat, cholesterol 37mg, protein 36.4g, carbohydrates 59.8g, **fiber 19.1g**, sugar 13.3g, sodium 76mg

TROPICAL TANGY FRUIT SALAD
Prep: 10 min.

2 navel oranges, white pith discarded, cut crosswise into 1/4 inch slices
4 bananas, peeled and cut into 1/2 inch slices
1 mango, peeled, pitted and chopped
1 Tbs. lime juice
1/4 cup honey
1 cup plain lowfat yogurt

Combine oranges, bananas and mangos in a salad bowl. Add lime juice and toss. Combine honey and yogurt in another bowl. Pour over fruit and toss before serving.

PER SERVING: calories 371, fat 2.1g, 5% calories from fat, cholesterol 4mg, protein 6.2g, carbohydrates 92.1g, **fiber 9.7g**, sugar 76.5g, sodium 48mg

CHICKEN AND BLACK
BEAN SAUTÉ
Prep: 10 min, Cook: 20 min

2 tsp. unsalted butter
2/3 cup onion, finely chopped
1 lb. boneless skinless chicken breast halves, cut into 1 inch
pieces
2 lbs. black beans, drained
3/4 tsp. turmeric
1/4 tsp. cayenne pepper
1/4 tsp. pepper
4 scallions, sliced
2 cups plain lowfat yogurt
4 white pitas, opened at one side and lightly toasted

Melt butter in a heavy nonstick skillet over medium high heat.
Sauté onion 5-7 minutes or until golden. Add chicken and
sauté 3-4 minutes or until chicken is lightly browned. Stir in
black beans, turmeric, cayenne and pepper and sauté 3-4
minutes. Reduce heat to medium low. Stir in half the scallions.
Sauté 2-3 minutes, stirring constantly until scallions are
softened. Remove from heat and stuff into pita breads.
Sprinkle with remaining scallions and a dollop of yogurt.

PER SERVING: calories 620, fat 6.9g, 10% calories from fat,
cholesterol 78mg, protein 53.0g, carbohydrates 85.2g, **fiber
18.9g**, sugar 20.7g, sodium 704mg

HEALTHY CAJUN BEANS AND RICE
Prep: 10 min, Cook: 15 min.

1 Tbs. vegetable oil
1/2 lb. turkey sausage, sliced into 1/2 inch thick slices
1 medium onion, chopped
1 medium green bell pepper, chopped
2 cloves garlic, minced
4-2/3 cups cooked rice
1 lb. canned kidney beans, drained and rinsed
1 lb. canned navy beans, drained and rinsed
3-1/2 cups canned stewed tomatoes, Cajun-style
1 tsp. oregano
1/2 tsp. hot pepper sauce
1 cup green onions, thinly sliced

Heat oil in large skillet over medium-high heat until hot. Add
sausage, onion, green pepper, and garlic. Cook, stirring 7-10
minutes, or until sausage is browned and onion is tender. Add
rice, kidney beans, navy beans, tomatoes, oregano, and hot
pepper sauce. Cook and stir 2-3 minutes more until well
blended and thoroughly heated. Sprinkle with green onions
and serve immediately.

PER SERVING: calories 695, fat 10.6g, 14% calories from
fat, cholesterol 35mg, protein 31.1g, carbohydrates 120.7g,
fiber 14.2g, sugar 17.1g, sodium 942mg

SPICY CUBAN CHICKEN

Prep: 15 min, Cook: 15 min, plus refrigeration time

2/3 cup nonfat Italian dressing
2 cloves garlic, minced
1/4 tsp. ground red pepper
11 ounces boneless, skinless chicken breasts, cut into 1/4 inch-thick strips
2 tsp. olive oil
1-1/4 medium green bell peppers, chopped
3/4 medium onion, chopped
3/4 tsp. oregano
1/4 tsp. ground black pepper
1/4 tsp. ground cumin
3 cups cooked rice
1-1/4 lbs. canned black beans, drained and rinsed
1-1/4 lbs. canned, diced tomatoes
3/4 tsp. fresh cilantro, chopped

Combine dressing, garlic, and red pepper in a glass measure or medium glass bowl. Place chicken in large glass bowl, pour dressing over chicken, cover and **refrigerate** 30-60 minutes (or overnight). Remove chicken from marinade, drain well, discard marinade.

Heat oil in large skillet over medium-high heat until hot. Add chicken, cook 5-7 minutes, stirring until chicken is slightly brown, spooning off any excess liquid. Add bell peppers, onion, oregano, pepper, and cumin. Cook, stirring 4-5 minutes or until vegetables are tender. Add rice, black beans, and tomatoes. Cook 2-3 minutes more, or until thoroughly heated.

Garnish with cilantro, serve immediately.

PER SERVING: calories 522, fat 6.5g, 11% calories from fat, cholesterol 66mg, protein 38.4g, carbohydrates 76.6g, **fiber 13.1g**, sugar 14.3g, sodium 596mg

BANANA DATE NUT SALAD IN PASTRY
Prep: 10 min, Cook: 10 min.

4 frozen puff pastry shells
2 bananas, peeled and cut into 1/2 inch slices
8 dates, pitted and chopped
1/4 cup chopped walnuts
1 tsp. lemon juice

Bake puff pastry shells according to package directions. Combine bananas, dates and walnuts in a mixing bowl. Sprinkle with lemon juice and toss. Just before serving, spoon fruit mixture into baked puff pastry shells.

PER SERVING: calories 574, fat 23.2g, 34% calories from fat, cholesterol 0mg, protein 7.2g, carbohydrates 92.6g, **fiber 13.1g**, sugar 56.0g, sodium 119mg

BLACK BEANS IN PITA POCKETS
Prep: 10 min, Marinate: 30 min.

1-1/2 lbs. canned black beans, rinsed and drained

2 Tbs. chopped pimento

2 Tbs. parsley

1 Tbs. plus 1 tsp. olive oil

2 Tbs. lemon juice

1-1/2 Tbs. water

1/4 tsp. dry mustard

1 clove garlic, minced

4 pita pocket breads, warm and cut in half

Combine beans, pimento and parsley in a salad bowl. Combine remaining ingredients, except pitas, in a jar with a tight-fitting lid. Add salt and pepper to taste. Shake vigorously. Pour dressing over beans. **Set aside** 30 minutes. Divide equally and stuff into pita breads.

PER SERVING: calories 366, fat 5.8g, 14% calories from fat, cholesterol 0mg, protein 16.0g, carbohydrates 63.1g, **fiber 13.3g**, sugar 7.2g, sodium 487mg

ZITI WITH BROCCOLI AND WHITE BEANS
Prep: 5 min, Cook: 10 min.

1/2 lb. ziti
2-2/3 cups broccoli florets
1-1/2 tsp. olive oil
2 cloves garlic, minced
1 cup dry white wine
14 ounces canned cannellini beans, drained and rinsed
1/4 cup grated Parmesan cheese

Cook pasta in a large pan of boiling water 10-12 minutes, or until al dente. During the last 2-3 minutes of cooking, add broccoli. Drain pasta and broccoli, set aside and keep warm. Heat oil in a heavy nonstick skillet over medium heat. Sauté garlic 1 minute, stirring constantly. Add wine and beans. Bring to a boil over high heat. Reduce heat to medium and cook about 5 minutes, until liquid is slightly reduced. Toss pasta and broccoli with sauce. Sprinkle on cheese and season with salt and pepper to taste. Toss again.

PER SERVING: calories 569, fat 5.3g, 8% calories from fat, cholesterol 4mg, protein 25.3g, carbohydrates 103.5g, **fiber 10.2g**, sugar 8.3g, sodium 125mg

SCAMPI WITH WHITE BEANS
Prep: 15 min, Cook: 15 min.

1 lb. asparagus, cut diagonally into 1 inch pieces
5 cloves garlic, minced
2 tsp. olive oil
2 tsp. margarine
1 lb. shrimp, peeled, deveined
2 cups tomatoes, chopped
1 lb. canned Great Northern beans, or navy beans, rinsed, drained
1/2 tsp. dried marjoram
1/2 tsp. dried basil leaves
1/2 tsp. dried rosemary leaves
2/3 cup low sodium chicken broth
2 tsp. cornstarch
1/2 lb. spinach fettuccine, cooked, hot
2 Tbs. grated Parmesan cheese, or fat-free grated Parmesan

Cook asparagus and garlic in oil and margarine in large skillet over medium heat 1-2 minutes. Add shrimp and cook until pink, 2-3 minutes. Add tomatoes, beans, and herbs; cook, covered, until tomatoes are wilted, 2-3 minutes. Mix chicken broth and cornstarch, stir into skillet. Cook over medium heat until thickened, stirring frequently. Season to taste with salt and pepper. Serve over fettuccine and sprinkle with cheese.

Variation: Substitute 1 lb. boneless, skinless chicken breast for the shrimp. Cut the chicken into 3/4 inch pieces; cook chicken in oil and margarine in large skillet over medium heat 3-4 minutes. Add asparagus and garlic; cook until chicken is no longer pink in the center, 2-3 minutes. Complete recipe as above.

PER SERVING: calories 513, fat 9.0g, 15% calories from fat, cholesterol 175mg, protein 43.4g, carbohydrates 68.2g, **fiber 13.3g**, sugar 8.3g, sodium 379mg

SWEET RASPBERRY AND BANANA SMOOTHIE
Prep: 5 min.

4 cups fresh raspberries
4 bananas
4 cups skim milk
3/4 cup vanilla lowfat yogurt
2 Tbs. plus 2 tsp. sugar

Combine all ingredients in a blender or food processor and process until smooth.

PER SERVING: calories 378, fat 2.5g, 6% calories from fat, cholesterol 7mg, protein 13.8g, carbohydrates 81.8g, **fiber 12.6g**, sugar 70.6g, sodium 158mg

CALIFORNIA CHICKEN AND BEANS
Prep: 10 min, Cook: 20 min.

1 lb. boneless, skinless chicken breasts

1 Tbs. vegetable oil

2 green onions, with tops, sliced

1/2 tsp. garlic, minced

1-3/4 cups low sodium chicken broth, fat-free

1/4 cup all purpose flour

1 lb. frozen mixed vegetables

1 lb. canned pinto beans, or kidney beans, drained and rinsed

7 ounces button mushrooms, drained

1 tsp. dried rosemary leaves

Cook chicken in oil in large saucepan over medium heat until browned, about 5 minutes. Add green onion and garlic and cook 1 minute. Combine chicken broth and flour; add to sauce pan. Add frozen vegetables, beans, mushrooms, and herbs and heat to boiling; reduce heat and simmer, covered, until chicken vegetables are tender, 8-10 minutes. Season to taste and salt and pepper.

This recipe can be prepared 1-2 days in advance; refrigerate, covered. Serve over cooked rice or noodles, if desired.

PER SERVING: calories 457, fat 9.9g, 19% calories from fat, cholesterol 99mg, protein 47.8g, carbohydrates 46.2g, **fiber 12.9g**, sugar 9.6g, sodium 259mg

BEAN AND CHEESE SANDWICHES
Prep: 5 min, Cook: 10 min.

1 lb. canned black beans, drained
1/4 cup recipe-ready crushed tomatoes
1/4 tsp. ground cumin
4 hoagy sandwich buns, cut in half lengthwise
3/4 cup shredded cheddar cheese
1 cup salsa

Preheat oven to 400°F. Combine beans, tomatoes and cumin in a blender or food processor. Process until smooth. Transfer to a heavy nonstick skillet over medium heat. Stir 2-3 minutes or until hot. Remove from heat and set aside. Remove a small amount of center of each bread half to make a shallow hollow and divide beans among sandwich halves. Sprinkle with cheese. Place sandwiches on a baking sheet and bake in oven about 5 minutes or until cheese is melted. Serve sandwiches with salsa.

PER SERVING: calories 595, fat 11.6g, 18% calories from fat, cholesterol 22mg, protein 25.0g, carbohydrates 97.2g, **fiber 12.2g**, sugar 11.6g, sodium 1280mg

TRI-COLORED TORTELLINI SALAD
Prep: 10 min, Cook: 10 min.

9 ounces fresh multicolored cheese tortellini
6 ounces marinated artichoke hearts, drained, marinade reserved
1 Tbs. balsamic vinegar
2 Tbs. fresh basil, slivered
9 ounces sun-dried tomatoes, prepared according to package directions, drained and chopped
1/4 cup black olives, sliced, drained
1 small head lettuce, torn

Cook tortellini in a large pan of boiling water 7 minutes, or until al dente. Drain and set aside. Combine reserved artichoke marinade, vinegar and basil in a bowl. Add tortellini, tomatoes, olives and artichokes. Season with salt to taste. Toss gently and serve on a bed of lettuce.

PER SERVING: calories 433, fat 11.1g, 21% calories from fat, cholesterol 24mg, protein 20.5g, carbohydrates 70.7g, **fiber 12.1g**, sugar 26.0g, sodium 1824mg

SMOKED TURKEY STUFFED PITAS
Prep: 10 min, Cook: 10 min.

1/4 cup lemon juice
1 Tbs. unsalted butter, cut into pieces
1 tsp. olive oil
1 red bell pepper, seeded and cut into 1/4 inch thin strips
1 lb. zucchini, cut into 1/4 inch thin strips
1-1/2 lbs. jicama, peeled and cut into 1/4 inch thin strips
3/4 lb. smoked turkey, cut into 1/2 inch cubes
2 Tbs. water
4 white pitas, cut in half crosswise

Bring lemon juice to a boil in a heavy non-reactive saucepan
over medium heat. Boil 2-3 minutes or until juice is reduced to
1 Tbs. Remove from heat and let stand 1 minute. Stir in butter
until it is incorporated. Heat oil in a wok or heavy nonstick
skillet over medium high heat. Add bell pepper, zucchini,
jicama and turkey and sauté 2-3 minutes. Add water and sauté
another 3-4 minutes or until vegetables are tender. Drizzle with
lemon butter. Season with salt and pepper to taste and toss.
Stuff pitas with sautéed turkey and vegetables.

PER SERVING: calories 369, fat 7.1g, 16% calories from fat,
cholesterol 43mg, protein 25.2g, carbohydrates 56.1g, **fiber
11.3g**, sugar 8.3g, sodium 1428mg

LENTIL CHICKEN SALAD

Prep: 10 min, Cook: 20 min, plus refrigeration time.

2/3 cup lentils
1-1/2 cups water
1/4 cup light mayonnaise
2 Tbs. green onions, chopped
1/8 tsp. hot red pepper sauce
1 cup cooked chicken, diced
1/2 cup celery, diced
1/2 cup cucumber, diced
1/4 cup green bell pepper, diced
2 ounces chopped pimento
4 cups mixed salad greens
1 Tbs. fresh parsley, chopped

Rinse lentils in cold water and drain. Bring water to a boil in a heavy nonstick pan over medium high heat. Reduce heat and add lentils. Cover and **simmer** about 20 minutes, or until lentils are just tender. Drain and **refrigerate** until cooled. Combine next 3 ingredients in a small bowl and mix well. Combine cooled lentils, chicken and next 4 ingredients in a medium bowl. Pour in dressing and mix gently. Cover and **refrigerate** at least 1 hour. To serve, arrange salad greens on individual plates and top with chicken salad. Sprinkle with parsley.

PER SERVING: calories 280, fat 12.6g, 40% calories from fat, cholesterol 33mg, protein 19.0g, carbohydrates 24.2g, **fiber 11.1g**, sugar 3.3g, sodium 105mg

ITALIAN VEGETABLE RICE SOUP
Prep: 5 min, Cook: 10 min.

1-1/2 quarts vegetable or chicken stock
2 carrots, peeled and diced
1 zucchini, diced
1 lb. canned Great Northern beans, undrained
1-1/2 cups quick cooking rice
1 tsp. Italian herb seasoning
1/4 cup grated Parmesan cheese

Bring stock and carrots to a boil in a saucepan over high heat.
Stir in next 4 ingredients. Cook about 5 minutes, until
vegetables are just tender. Serve sprinkled with Parmesan.

PER SERVING: calories 331, fat 3.1g, 8% calories from fat,
cholesterol 4mg, protein 15.6g, carbohydrates 61.2g, **fiber
10.7g**, sugar 5.2g, sodium 525mg

STIR-FRIED BLACKEYES AND PORK
Prep: 10 min, Cook: 20 min.

1/2 lb. boneless pork tenderloin chops, cut into 1-1/2 inch-
thick strips
2-3/4 green onions, with tops, sliced
2 cloves garlic, minced
2 tsp. vegetable oil
1-1/3 cups broccoli florets

10 ounces canned black-eyed beans, or pinto beans, drained
and rinsed
1/4 cup plus 3 Tbs. reduced-sodium beef broth
1/4 cup plus 3 Tbs. low sodium soy sauce
2-3/4 tsp. cornstarch
1 cup halved cherry tomatoes
2 cups hot cooked rice

Stir-fry pork, green onion, and garlic in oil in wok or large
skillet over high heat until pork is browned, 3-5 minutes. Add
broccoli and stir-fry 2-3 minutes. Add beans and cook,
covered, over medium heat until broccoli is crisp-tender, 3-4
minutes.

Mix beef broth, soy sauce, and cornstarch; add to skillet and
heat to boiling. Boil, stirring constantly, until thickened, about
1 minute. Add tomatoes; cook 1-2 minutes longer. Season to
taste with pepper. Serve over rice.

Note: You can substitute cooked Chinese egg noodles for the
rice, if desired.

PER SERVING: calories 526, fat 6.2g, 10% calories from fat,
cholesterol 36mg, protein 35.9g, carbohydrates 83.4g, **fiber
10.6g**, sugar 11.8g, sodium 1093mg

BASIC MICROWAVE WINTER SQUASH
Prep: 5 min, Cook: 10 min.

4 cups winter squash, de-seeded and sliced into 1/4 inch slices
1 cup water

Place winter squash in microwave-safe dish. Add water. Cover and **cook** on high for 10-13 minutes, or until tender when pierced with a fork.

PER SERVING: calories 115, fat 0.3g, 2% calories from fat, cholesterol 0mg, protein 2.3g, carbohydrates 29.9g, **fiber 9.0g**, sugar 7.2g, sodium 10mg

MOGUL BEEF AND BEANS
Prep: 10 min, Cook: 15 min.

1/2 tsp. ground cumin
1/2 tsp. ground cardamom
1 Tbs. plus 1 tsp. olive oil
2 onions, cut into 1/2 inch pieces
2 cups Italian style peeled tomatoes, drained and sliced
1 lb. canned black beans, drained
4 top sirloin steaks, about 1/4 lb. each

Combine cumin, cardamom, and salt and pepper to taste in a bowl and set aside. Heat half the oil in a heavy nonstick skillet over medium heat. Sauté onions 4 minutes, stirring occasionally. Stir in tomatoes, spice mixture, and beans. Cover and simmer 6 minutes, or until onions are tender. Transfer onion mixture to a platter and keep warm. Wipe skillet clean with a paper towel. Add remaining oil and heat over medium high heat. Sauté steaks 3-4 minutes per side for medium-done meat. Season with salt and pepper to taste. Serve steaks over tomato sauce and beans.

PER SERVING: calories 455, fat 15.3g, 30% calories from fat, cholesterol 112mg, protein 47.3g, carbohydrates 32.0g, **fiber 10.2g**, sugar 11.9g, sodium 372mg

TUSCAN WHITE BEANS AND RICE

Prep: 10 min, Cook: 20 min.

2 tsp. olive oil
1/2 lb. boneless, skinless chicken breasts, cut into 1/4 inch-thick strips
3/4 medium onion, chopped
2 cloves garlic, minced
5 ounces fresh spinach leaves, washed, stems removed, torn
1-1/4 cups canned diced tomatoes, drained
3 cups cooked rice
1-1/4 lbs. canned navy beans, or canned Great Northern beans, drained and rinsed
1-1/4 tsp. Italian herb seasoning
1 Tbs. plus 1 tsp. red wine vinegar
1 Tbs. plus 1 tsp. dry sherry

1/4 tsp. ground black pepper

1/2 cup grated Parmesan cheese

Heat oil in large skilled over medium-high heat until hot. Add chicken onion, and garlic; cook 7-10 minutes or until chicken is slightly browned and onion is tender. Add spinach and tomatoes. Cook 3-4 minutes more or until spinach is wilted and tomatoes are simmering. Add rice, navy beans, Italian seasoning, vinegar, sherry and pepper. Cook and stir 3-4 minutes more until thoroughly heated. Sprinkle with Parmesan cheese.

You can substitute 13 ounces frozen spinach leaves, thawed and drained, for fresh spinach, if desired.

PER SERVING: calories 541, fat 8.1g, 14% calories from fat, cholesterol 55mg, protein 37.5g, carbohydrates 78.4g, **fiber 9.9g**, sugar 11.0g, sodium 365mg

SOUTHWESTERN BEEF SALAD
Prep: 15 min, Cook: 15 min.

1 lb. lean ground beef

1/2 cup onions, chopped

1 Tbs. chili powder

2 tsp. dried oregano

1/2 tsp. ground cumin

1 cup canned red kidney beans, drained and rinsed

1 lb. canned chickpeas, drained and rinsed

1 medium tomato, diced
2 cups lettuce
1/2 cup cheddar cheese

Cook ground beef and onion in a skillet over medium-high heat until beef is no longer pink, about 10 to 12 minutes. Drain. Stir in chili powder, oregano, and cumin. Cook for 1 minute. Mix in beans, chickpeas, and tomato. Portion lettuce onto serving plates. Top with grated cheese. Then top with beef mixture.

PER SERVING: calories 432, fat 17.9g, 37% calories from fat, cholesterol 56mg, protein 35.7g, carbohydrates 32.6g, **fiber 10.3g**, sugar 3.9g, sodium 311mg

SPICY ITALIAN SKI TEAM SOUP
Prep: 10 min, Cook: 20 min.

1/3 cup onions, chopped
1/3 cup green bell pepper, chopped
3/4 tsp. garlic, minced
1/4 tsp. crushed red pepper
1-1/4 tsp. olive oil
1 cup reduced-sodium beef broth
1 cup water
11 ounces canned kidney beans, drained and rinsed
1-1/4 cups canned Italian style stewed tomatoes
11 ounces frozen Italian-style vegetable combination
3/4 tsp. dried basil leaves
1/2 cup small shell pasta

2/3 cup spinach leaves, loosely packed

Sauté onion, pepper, garlic, and red pepper in oil in large saucepan until tender, 3-4 minutes. Stir in beef broth, water, beans, tomatoes, Italian vegetables, and basil; heat to boiling. Add pasta and **simmer**, uncovered, until vegetables and pasta are tender, about 10 minutes. Stir spinach into soup; simmer 1-2 minutes. Season to taste with salt and pepper. If desired, add a teaspoon of prepared pesto sauce into each bowl of soup.

You can substitute frozen chopped onion, green pepper, and prepared garlic. You can prepare soup 1-2 days in advance; refrigerate, covered.

PER SERVING: calories 230, fat 2.4g, 9% calories from fat, cholesterol 0mg, protein 11.9g, carbohydrates 43.1g, **fiber 9.2g**, sugar 7.4g, sodium 499mg

FRESH PINEAPPLE FRUIT SALAD
Prep: 10 min, plus chilling time.

1 whole pineapple
1 papaya, peeled, seeded, cut into chunks
1/4 lb. seedless grapes
1 apple, peeled cored and cut into chunks
1/4 cup pecan halves
1 banana, sliced
1/4 cup lime juice
1 lime, quartered, as garnish

Cut pineapple lengthwise into quarters. Cut away and discard core. Remove pineapple flesh by carefully cutting between it and outer skin of pineapple to use the shell for a salad bowl. Cut pineapple into chunks and combine with remaining ingredients, except lime wedges, in a bowl. Gently toss and **chill** if desired. Serve fruit salad in a pineapple shell topped with lime garnish.

PER SERVING: calories 299, fat 6.7g, 18% calories from fat, cholesterol 0mg, protein 3.1g, carbohydrates 65.5g, **fiber 8.4g**, sugar 50.8g, sodium 7mg

SQUASH AND YAM SOUP
Prep: 15 min, Cook: 20 min.

2 lbs. butternut squash, peeled, seeded and cut into 1 inch pieces
3/4 lb. yams, peeled and cut into 1 inch pieces
1 Tbs. unsalted butter
1 onion, chopped
2 cloves garlic, minced
1 Tbs. fresh ginger, peeled and minced
1/2 tsp. cinnamon
1/4 tsp. ground ginger
1/8 tsp. red pepper flakes
4 cups vegetable stock
2 Tbs. pure maple syrup
2 Tbs. orange marmalade

Place squash and yams in a steamer basket over boiling water. Cover saucepan and **steam** 20 minutes or until tender. Remove steamer basket and set aside. Melt butter in a heavy nonstick skillet over medium high heat. Sauté onions 7-8 minutes or until golden brown. Stir in garlic and fresh ginger and sauté 1 minute. Stir in cinnamon, ground ginger and chili pepper flakes. Add half the stock to skillet, stirring with a wooden spoon to deglaze. Working in batches, purée onion mixture, squash, yams and maple syrup in a blender or food processor until smooth. Transfer purée to a saucepan. Add remaining stock, salt and pepper to taste. Cook until heated throughout. Serve with a dollop of orange marmalade.

PER SERVING: calories 310, fat 4.0g, 11% calories from fat, cholesterol 8mg, protein 4.6g, carbohydrates 69.6g, **fiber 12.0g**, sugar 22.2g, sodium 499mg

GERMAN BEAN AND SAUSAGE SOUP
Prep: 10 min, Cook: 20 min.

3/4 tsp. oil

1/3 cup onion, chopped

2/3 cup carrots, sliced

2/3 cup potato, peeled, cubed

2 Tbs. plus 2 tsp. fresh parsley, chopped

1/4 tsp. dried marjoram leaves (optional)

1 cup beef stock

5 ounces smoked turkey kielbasa, cut into 1/2 inch slices

10 ounces canned Great Northern beans, undrained

9 ounces canned cut green beans, undrained

Heat oil in a saucepan over medium heat. Sauté onion 4-5 minutes, stirring frequently, until tender. Add carrots and next 4 ingredients. Season with salt and pepper to taste. Bring to a boil. Reduce heat to low, cover and **simmer** about 15 minutes or until vegetables are tender. Add sausage and beans. Cook until thoroughly heated.

PER SERVING: calories 192, fat 4.3g, 19% calories from fat, cholesterol 23mg, protein 13.8g, carbohydrates 26.5g, **fiber 7.6g**, sugar 5.3g, sodium 694mg

MONDAY-NITE TURKEY & BEANS OVER RICE
Prep: 10 min, Cook: 20 min.

2 cups water or chicken stock
1 cup white rice
1 Tbs. vegetable oil
3/4 cup celery, chopped
4 scallions, chopped
2 cloves garlic, minced
1/3 cup red wine
1 lb. canned kidney beans, rinsed and drained
2 cups cooked turkey, diced
1/4 cup dried oregano, crumbled
1/8 tsp. pepper
1-1/2 cups water
1 Tbs. cornstarch, blended with 1 Tbs. water
3 Tbs. lite soy sauce

Boil water in a medium saucepan over high heat. Stir in rice and immediately reduce heat to low. Cover and **simmer** 20 minutes or until rice is tender and liquid is absorbed. Heat oil in a saucepan over medium heat. Stir-fry celery, scallions and garlic 2 minutes. Stir in next 6 ingredients, cover pan and bring to a boil. Reduce heat to low and **simmer** 15 minutes. Stir cornstarch mixture into pan. Bring to a boil and cook, stirring, 1 minute. Remove from heat and stir in soy sauce. Serve over rice.

PER SERVING: calories 512, fat 11.6g, 21% calories from fat, cholesterol 57mg, protein 31.1g, carbohydrates 66.8g, **fiber 9.0g**, sugar 4.9g, sodium 579mg

FRESH FRUIT SALAD
Prep: 15 min.

2 large peaches, sliced
2 cups blueberries, picked over
2 firm bananas, peeled and sliced
1/2 lb. Bing cherries, halved and pitted
2 cups fresh strawberries, hulled and halved
1/4 cup sugar
1/4 cup Grand Marnier or other orange liqueur (optional)
2 cups plain or vanilla nonfat yogurt

Combine fruit with sugar and Grand Marnier in a large bowl. Toss and transfer to a serving bowl. Serve with yogurt.

PER SERVING: calories 336, fat 2.5g, 6% calories from fat, cholesterol 2mg, protein 10.8g, carbohydrates 76.3g, **fiber 8.7g**, sugar 65.2g, sodium 100mg

CHICKEN SAUSALITO
Prep: 10 min, Cook: 15 min.

1 vegetable cooking spray
1/2 lb. boneless, skinless chicken breasts, cut into 3/4 inch pieces
1/2 cup onion, chopped
1 tsp. garlic, minced
1 lb. canned black beans or red kidney beans, rinsed, drained
2/3 cup tomatoes, chopped
3 Tbs. salsa, mild or hot
1/2 cup lowfat sour cream
3 cups cooked rice, warm

Spray large skillet with cooking spray; heat over medium heat until hot. Sauté chicken, onion, and garlic until chicken is cooked, 5-8 minutes. Sprinkle chicken with flour and cook 1 minute longer. Stir in beans, tomato, salsa, and sour cream. Cook until hot, 1-2 minutes. Season to taste with salt and pepper. Spoon chicken mixture over rice. Serve with the garnish or your choice (chopped avocado, sliced green onions, and/or finely chopped cilantro or parsley).

PER SERVING: calories 434, fat 5.4g, 11% calories from fat, cholesterol 58mg, protein 30.8g, carbohydrates 63.8g, **fiber 9.2g**, sugar 8.7g, sodium 220mg

TOMATO BEAN SANDWICH
Prep: 10 min.

3/4 cup canned black beans, drained and mashed
2 Tbs. plus 2 tsp. peanut butter
2 Tbs. plus 2 tsp. sun dry tomato spread
8 slices whole wheat bread, toasted if desired
4 lettuce leaves

Combine first 3 ingredients in a bowl. Spread mixture on one slice of bread and top with lettuce and remaining bread slice.

PER SERVING: calories 314, fat 8.6g, 25% calories from fat, cholesterol 0mg, protein 11.9g, carbohydrates 47.8g, **fiber 8.3g**, sugar 6.8g, sodium 463mg

CHICKEN AND BEAN BONANZA
Prep: 10 min, Cook: 15 min.

1 cup onion, chopped
1/3 cup green or red bell pepper, chopped
3/4 tsp. garlic, minced
2 tsp. vegetable oil
1/2 lb. boneless, skinless chicken breasts, cut into small pieces
3/4 tsp. ground cumin
1/2 tsp. ground cinnamon

10 ounces canned navy beans, or garbanzo beans, drained and
rinsed
10 ounces canned red beans, or kidney beans, drained and
rinsed
10 ounces Italian-style stewed tomatoes, undrained
2 Tbs. plus 2 tsp. raisins

Sauté onion, pepper, and garlic in oil in medium saucepan 2-3
minutes. Add chicken, cumin, and cinnamon; cook over
medium-high heat until chicken is lightly browned, about 3-4
minutes. Add beans, tomatoes, and raisins; heat to boiling.
Reduce heat and simmer, uncovered, until slightly thickened,
about 5- 8 minutes. Season to taste with salt and pepper.

Additional tips: Frozen chopped onion and green pepper, and
prepared garlic can be used. The dish is delicious served over
cooked rice, couscous, or pasta. Can be prepared 1-2 days in
advance; refrigerate, covered.

PER SERVING: calories 321, fat 4.9g, 14% calories from fat,
cholesterol 48mg, protein 27.9g, carbohydrates 41.6g, **fiber
7.9g**, sugar 16.2g, sodium 256mg

RICE WITH PEAS AND PARMESAN
Prep: 10 min, Cook: 20 min.

1 Tbs. unsalted butter
3 Tbs. onion, minced
1 cup short grain rice
2 cups chicken stock

1 lb. frozen baby peas, thawed

1/4 cup grated Parmesan cheese

Melt butter in a heavy saucepan over medium heat. Sauté
onion 3 minutes or until softened. Add rice and sauté 2
minutes, stirring constantly. Stir in stock. Increase heat to high
and bring to a boil. Immediately reduce heat to low. Cover
sauccpan and **simmer** 10 minutes. Add peas to saucepan,
without stirring, and steam another 5-10 minutes, or until rice
is tender and liquid is absorbed. Stir in Parmesan, and salt and
pepper to taste.

PER SERVING: calories 336, fat 5.5g, 15% calories from fat,
cholesterol 11mg, protein 13.6g, carbohydrates 57.1g, **fiber
7.8g**, sugar 7.3g, sodium 573mg

BANANA RAISIN SALAD

Prep: 5 min.

4 bananas

8 lettuce leaves

1/4 cup mayonnaise type salad dressing

1 tsp. cinnamon

1/2 cup raisins

Split bananas. Arrange on a bed of lettuce leaves. Spread
mayonnaise type salad dressing down centers of banana halves.
Sprinkle with cinnamon and dot with raisins.

PER SERVING: calories 284, fat 5.9g, 17% calories from fat,
cholesterol 4mg, protein 2.8g, carbohydrates 61.6g, **fiber
5.5g**, sugar 50.8g, sodium 110mg

BERRY-BANANA-PEACH SMOOTHIE

Prep: 5 min.

4 cups lowfat blueberry yogurt
2 cups peach nectar
4 ripe bananas

Mix all ingredients in a blender and then serve.

PER SERVING: calories 478, fat 3.7g, 7% calories from fat, cholesterol 10mg, protein 12.8g, carbohydrates 105.1g, **fiber 5.2g**, sugar 95.5g, sodium 154mg

LEMONY GREEN BEANS

Prep: 5 min, Cook: 10 min.

1 tsp. sesame seeds
1-1/2 lbs. green beans, thawed if frozen
1/2 cup chicken stock
1/8 tsp. salt (optional)
2 tsp. lemon juice

Toast sesame seeds in a heavy nonstick skillet over medium heat, about 3 minutes, shaking pan constantly until seeds are browned and have popped. Add green beans, stock, salt and pepper to taste. Cover skillet and cook 7-8 minutes or until green beans are tender and liquid is evaporated. Remove from heat. Stir in lemon juice before serving.

PER SERVING: calories 63, fat 0.8g, 10% calories from fat, cholesterol 0mg, protein 3.9g, carbohydrates 12.6g, **fiber 5.9g**, sugar 4.6g, sodium 108mg

CHICKEN WITH VEGETABLE MARINARA
Prep: 10 min, Cook: 10 min.

1 lb. eggplant, peeled and cubed
1 red bell pepper, seeded and cubed
1 large zucchini, peeled and cubed
1/4 cup chicken or vegetable stock
4 cups purchased spaghetti sauce
1 Tbs. olive oil
1-1/4 lbs. boneless skinless chicken breast halves
1/4 cup lemon juice
4 slices French bread, toasted
2 Tbs. grated Parmesan cheese

Turn on broiler. Combine first 4 ingredients in a heavy nonstick skillet over medium high heat. Cover skillet and simmer 4-5 minutes, or until vegetables are tender and liquid is almost evaporated. Stir in spaghetti sauce and cook until mixture is heated throughout. Set aside and keep warm.

While sauce is cooking, brush chicken with oil and season with pepper to taste. Arrange on a broiler pan and broil 4 minutes per side until chicken is opaque throughout. Remove chicken from broiler and immediately drizzle with lemon juice. Serve chicken on toast. Spoon sauce over chicken, sprinkle with Parmesan and serve.

PER SERVING: calories 458, fat 12.1g, 24% calories from fat, cholesterol 84mg, protein 42.0g, carbohydrates 45.2g, **fiber 8.7g**, sugar 6.6g, sodium 1371mg

CHILLED PEA SOUP
Prep: 10 min, Cook: 5 min, plus refrigeration time.

10 ounces frozen peas
2 green onions, chopped
2 cups low sodium chicken broth
1/2 tsp. dried dill
1 cup plain lowfat yogurt

Place peas, onions, 1/4 cup of the chicken broth and dill in a heavy nonstick pan over medium high heat. Cover and cook 5-6 minutes, or until peas are tender. Remove from heat and cool. Stir in remaining chicken broth. Working in batches, transfer pea mixture to a blender or food processor and process until smooth. Pour blended mixture into a bowl and repeat process until whole mixture is puréed. Cover and **refrigerate** until chilled. Just before serving, whisk yogurt into pea soup. Pour into individual serving bowls and top with an extra spoonful of yogurt, if desired.

PER SERVING: calories 130, fat 2.2g, 15% calories from fat, cholesterol 6mg, protein 9.1g, carbohydrates 20.3g, **fiber 5.3g**, sugar 12.3g, sodium 162mg

CHINESE STEAMED FISH

Prep: 10 min, Marinate: 30 min, Cook: 10 min.

2 Tbs. lite soy sauce

1 Tbs. Asian sesame oil

3/4 tsp. fresh ginger, grated

3 Tbs. rice vinegar

1/4 cup plus 2 Tbs. orange juice

3/4 tsp. orange rind, grated

1-1/2 lbs. cod fillets or white fish, about 3/4 inch thick, rinsed
with cold water

1-1/2 cups mushrooms, sliced

4 scallions, cut into 1 inch pieces

1-1/2 cups snow peas, cut into 1 inch pieces

1-1/2 cups carrots, sliced

Combine first 6 ingredients in a nonreactive bowl. **Marinate**
30 minutes. Drain marinade and transfer to a small saucepan
over medium high heat. Bring to a simmer and set aside.
Arrange fish on a steamer tray. Place tray over boiling water.
Cover and steam 2 minutes. Add remaining ingredients and
steam another 5 minutes until fish flakes easily and vegetables
are crisp-tender. Pour sauce over individual portions just
before serving.

PER SERVING: calories 255, fat 5.2g, 18% calories from fat,
cholesterol 73mg, protein 34.9g, carbohydrates 16.8g, **fiber
5.5g**, sugar 9.0g, sodium 398mg

Made in the USA
Lexington, KY
15 October 2014